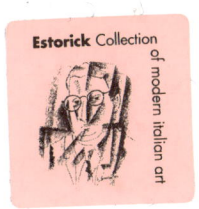

The Evolution of Imagination

Part 1.

THE NIGHTMARE OF SLEEP

Roger Cliffe-Thompson

First Published 2013 by The Cloister House Press

Copyright © 2013, Roger Cliffe-Thompson

The right of Roger Cliffe-Thompson to be identified as the author of this work has been asserted by him in accordance with the Copyright, Designs and Patents act 1988.

All rights reserved. No part of this book may be reproduced, stored in a retrieval system, or transmitted in any form or by any means, electronic, mechanical, photocopying, recording or otherwise, without the prior written permission of the author.

British library Cataloguing- in- Publication Data
British library CIP record is available

ISBN 978-1-909465-02-2

Typeset in Times new Roman.

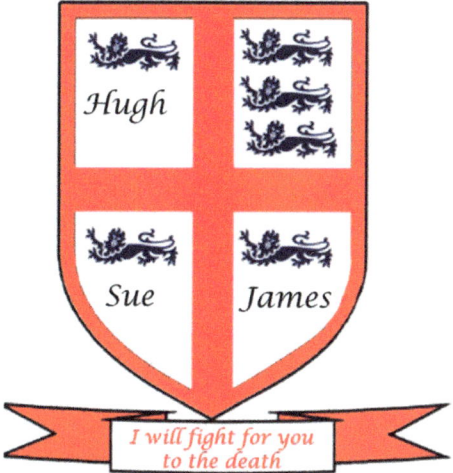

For Hugh, Sue, James and Coco, our Burmese,
who stole our hearts for twenty five years.

CONTENTS

Homo imaginus	1.
Time Lords	2.
The illusion of a free society	3-4.
Imagination-survival of the fittest	5.
Imagination-victim of prejudice	6-7.
Nature is obsolete	7-8.

THE BIOLOGICAL JOURNEY
Imagination begats imagination	10-11.
Cerebral v biological	12.
Voluntary termination!	13.

THE NIGHTMARE OF SLEEP
The unknown assailant	15.
Making sense out of nonsense	16-17
Sleep does not suddenly evolve ...	18-19.
Physician heal thyself	20.

THIS IS YOUR BRAIN SPEAKING
Electrical activity generated by the brain.	22.
Types of brain waves	23-24-25.
Sleep Spindles	26.
Strategy when studying for exams	27.
K-complex and sound waves	28.
The real purpose of sleep	29.

THE SLEEP CYCLE
Sleep cycle framework	31-32-33.
Paradoxical sleep	34.
24 stages of sleep chart	36.
REM sleep in animals	38.
Sleep is over 250 million years old!	38.
Origins of our REM sleep	39.
Flip-flop v Fusion	41.
REM sleep in mammals	42.
REM napping	43-44.
Hemispherical sleep	45.
Function of REM sleep	47.
REM leakage	49.
Interaction of SWS and REM	50.
Seep cycle mechanism (chart)	51.

Each night we fight for our lives	52.
Eye movement during communication	56-58.

IS SLEEP THE DEATH OF EACH DAYS LIFE?   60.

Each day's sanity is the insanity of dreams	61.
Daydreaming is an active regulated process	62.
Daydreaming and Alpha waves	63.
Why do we remember dreams?	64.
Dreams in animals	65.
Does an animal on its own body	66.
Defragging the brain	67.
Cognitive Youtube	68.
Mirror image of dreaming	69.

ILLUSTRATIONS

Iron Lungs	4.
Russian butcher- Russian shoe shop	5.
Foetal image - Music for deaf people	10.
Beta waves	23.
Apha-Theta waves	24.
Delta waves - Sleep spindles	25.
Memory card on pillow	27.
K-complex and soundwave	28.
Sleep cycle framework -diagram	31.
REM sleep	34.
Sleeping like a log	35.
24 stages of sleep-diagram	36.
Animal eye markings	43.
Lions in REM sleep	46.
Sleep cycle mechanism- diagram	51.
Eye movement during communication	55.

* Images on page 4-5 are unattributable, whilst every effort has been made to trace their authors I regret I have as yet not managed to do so. If any reader knows who they belong to I would be grateful if they could contact me so I can credit their photographs.
* Memory card on pillow, idea by Alan Dunn.
* Cover courtesy of NASA
* Sleeping like a log, Simon Turton
* All other images including front back cover have been created by C-T Blackmore. Animal photographs were taken on a family trip to Chester Zoo who are doing a brilliant job with wildlife conservation. Well worth a visit, especially to the Bat Cave!

Acknowledgements

I wish to express my sincere thanks to my readers, all personal friends, who have been extremely helpful and supportive during the evolution of this book:
To:
David J. Costello - award winning poet: Frank Diamand - Holocaust survivor who became one of the world's top fifty filmmakers: Alan Dunn - Lecturer in Contemporary Art, Leeds Metropolitan University: Dr Tanya Garrett - Dr and Clinical Psychologist with a great sense of humour: Paul Howell - Energy Advisor who was recently awarded Bsc hons 1st Class from the Open University and if that doesn't put him amongst life's achievers, I don't know what does.
Alistair Morrison BSc (Hons) Ecology - retired Environment Protection Officer who has protected the environment from me for the last forty years, taking me fishing all over Scotland: Christine Morrison- Alistair's long suffering (from me), wife and our true friend. Baden Prince Jnr, 'me mate' since we first met in a squat in Amsterdam and who quite rightly fell asleep whilst reading this book. Annemarie de Wildt - Conservator Amsterdam Museum, who cast one eagle eye over the original and her instant observations prompted the first change of many.
Also to Professor Ray Bull, for his enthusiastic help and support and kindly agreeing to write the foreword: Alan Dunn who gets another mention because without his practical help and encouragement I could never have produced this book: Phil Cantlay, borne the same day in the same ward, has literally been my lifelong friend and always enthusiastic about what I'm up to: Si Turton a young man I helped raise for twelve years and who has such a zest for life, he always cheers me up: Miles at Choir Press who is the nicest person always willing to help with good advice.
Finally in recognition of some truly inspiring individuals who have let me share their friendship; 'M', now a ninety eight year old Scottish Country Dance instructor on Flinders Island, who has had the greatest influence on our lives: Billy Moon a brilliant 'Imagineer' who found happiness in Ethiopia: Peter Telford one of lifes gentleman who has the amazing ability to get the best out of everybody: Tony Myers who gave us courage: Barry Fitton who never gives up and my great friend and mentor, Dr Bob Hogg, who taught me how to think.

Covers designed by C-T Blackmore and front Cover Image Credit: NASA; ESA; G. Illingworth, D. Magee, and P. Oesch, University of California, Santa Cruz; R. Bouwens, Leiden University; and the HUDF09 Team

Foreword

A considerable number of years ago I had the pleasure of first meeting the author of this book (Roger Cliffe-Thompson) when I was working at an Open University summer school on 'The Biological Bases of Behaviour'. Each week a new cohort of students arrived and we academic staff took turns regarding who lectured on which topics.
One of the topics was 'The Bases of Illusions', for which slides were provided in a carousel. Each slide presented a well known illusion which the lecturer had to explain to the dozens of students in the audience. To the end of this presentation I usually added some of my own slides that I thought would be even more interesting – the effects of which I hypothesised might help people with disfigured/damaged faces not appear so 'unusual'. One student greatly enthused about my slides and afterwards talked to me animatedly about them at length.

This was Roger, who described to me (given his wealth of experience then as a hair stylist) how he had styled/cut women's hair so as to achieve similar visual effects. He was probably the most imaginative student I had ever met.

In this new book Roger demonstrates his very unusual combination of creativity and scientific appreciation. In the many years that I have known him I have often thought that Roger must have two brains – one of a factual scientist and the other of an imaginative artist.

I strongly urge you to read this book, whether you (mostly) like science or you (mostly) like the arts. It will stretch your mind, as it did mine.

Professor Ray Bull DSc, FBPsS, FAPS

Homo imaginus.

When they come to write the history of eternity, Imagination will be classed as the most powerful tool ever created. It is a gift of such awesome potential that it will not only defeat nature but enable mankind to spread far beyond the outermost planets and perhaps stand full square before the face of their God.

Einstein said, "Imagination is more important than knowledge." For it was imagination that allowed him to ride a light wave to formulate the world's most famous equation $E=mc2$. His fantastical journey is only one shining example of the multitude of extraordinary successes achieved by this incredible 'accident' of evolution but perhaps its most extraordinary achievement of all is us...Homo imaginus"

Time Lords

Every time you touch your forehead you are less than seven millimetres away from a biological computer with more processing power than all the world's computers linked together. Its main function is to run a unique application called 'Imagination' which allows us, Homo sapiens, to live in two coexisting worlds, both the physical and the virtual, simultaneously. Imagination is the hidden force that controls every aspect of our life, for we are all inseparably bound to our very own 'multi-dimensional virtual-reality processor'.

On the face of it Imagination is a simple combination of two processes - the first is the ability to select a memory 'before' an event and the second is to be able to 'manipulate' it together with other memories, into a logical sequence, to predict an outcome

Yet this simple ability allows each of us to become a Time Lord, constantly travelling between the past, the present and the future, in less than the blink of an eye. Imagination is our very own subliminal problem solver, constantly running in the background to provide answers to 'what if' scenarios enabling us to mentally assess consequences, without having to hurt ourselves in the physical world, something no other member of the animal kingdom can do.

Imagination feeds on Imagination growing exponentially so who knows where it will lead, are we at the dawn of virtual telepathy? Will Imagination physically change us again as it has already? Will Iit prove to be the saviour of our species or open a Pandora's Box of seismic proportions?

Time will eventually tell but for now perhaps the only hope we have of unravelling the future is if we start by tracing the incredible evolutionary steps which led us to acquire this wonderful gift.

'The Nightmare of Sleep' is part one of the 'Evolution of Imagination' which attempts to define; what imagination is, how it functions, and trace its unique biological development in us, the Universe's first Time Lords.

The illusion of a free society

Sad isn't it every day you are acting out somebody else's Imagination. Someone who may be long dead, you have never met or even like but sure as eggs their thoughts are still controlling your behaviour. By reading this book you are not only indulging in my imagination but Gutenberg's as well. It is said that Gutenberg's idea came to him like 'a ray of light' - a perfect summation of the speed and brilliance of Imagination.

For without it, you and I would not be interacting like this. Further, by continuously using the product of his imagination his invention lives on and will still 'Kindle' your imagination long after his physical self produced countless generations of worms. Then Bill Gates arrived enabling me to become Guttenberg and produce this text at home, in a space one metre square, with hosts of imagined computer worms waiting to destroy it.

Not only are we living out Guttenberg's imagination, but a host of others and they all collaborate to limit our activities. The buildings we live in, work in, get educated in, play sport in, 'compute' in (surely now the ultimate opiate of the masses), have all been imagined by an architect. The way we behave in each area is further constrained by a co-operative of sub-imagineers who invent procedures to dictate how we live our lives in the minutest detail. Try straying into a bus lane, parking on a yellow line or inadvertently overstaying on a pay and display machine. Vengeance is swift and still uses Guttenberg's imagination in the form of an officious letter which further controls you by exhorting "You must not ignore this notice... or it may result in a County Court order against you and a warrant for your arrest." No wonder we are becoming a nation of nervous drivers?

Who hasn't suffered from 'redundancy shock', the result of an accountant who conceived the concept of 'down-sizing', now called 'right-sizing', or the politicians who visualise the 'harmonisation' of departments in Public Services. Not very harmonious for those who lose their jobs. But it doesn't end there; my wallpaper; my furniture; my entertainment, etc, are all the physical manifestation of someone else's imagination.

We live cocooned inside Imagination's embrace; films; TV; books; advertising, all created in virtually reality by someone else's brain and just as the physical necessity for wearing clothes has been subverted by fashion's logo. Imagination is the Homo sapiens brand. The only contribution I can make is that I nominally have a choice as to whose imagination I select and to what extent I indulge it. But even then choice is limited by my financial means and what is available to me at the time.

If I wish to travel I must subject myself to the constraints of the Motorway designer, the Rail timetabler, the easyJet flight scheduler, etc. Who all physically manipulate my behaviour and make me conform to their rules and regulations at the micro as well as the macro level.

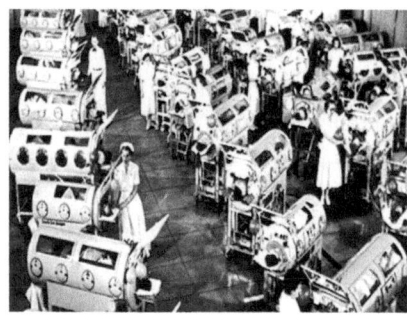 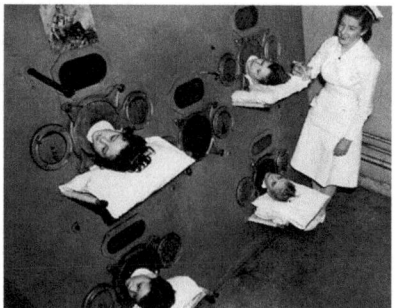

Iron lungs in USA last century - unattributed

For example; I have to find a suitable coin before I can use a supermarket trolley; discover when and where I can't use my mobile phone; desperately cram hand luggage into one of those absurd metal containers to see if I will be allowed to carry it onto a plane.
The list of constraints is virtually inexhaustible, we are bound tighter than any Gulliver by the Imagination of others yet live under the illusion that we live in a free society.

Like evolution - Ideas develop to their maximum efficiency and then become obsolete. Giant leaps in human development correlate neatly with society's willingness at the time to adapt to new ideas and new technology. This holds true from the Stone Age tools to the internal combustion engine.

Recently I attended a medical convention and an eminent clinician said, "The development in medicine in the past ten years is greater than the history of all medical discoveries put together."
This took me back to my childhood days in Whiston Hospital near Liverpool where I was incarcerated at the age of seven with Pneumonia. Imagine my astonishment when I saw what appeared to be a young boys head protruding from a massive metal cylinder. As soon as I was allowed out of bed I went to investigate and met Alan who gave me a cheery greeting through a car's rear view mirror screwed into the metal.
A Polio victim, he rested inside an Iron Lung (invented in 1927, by Philip Drinker and Louis Agassiz Shaw at Harvard University), which maintained his respiration artificially for a couple of weeks until he could breathe independently.

Iron Lungs reached their zenith 25 years later in 1952 when the USA experienced its worst polio epidemic with 58,000 cases.

Imagination - survival of the fittest

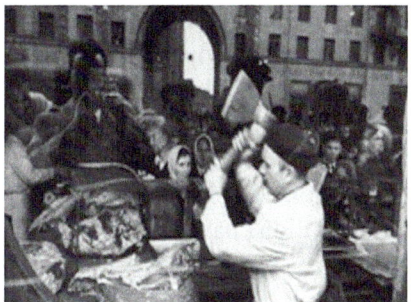 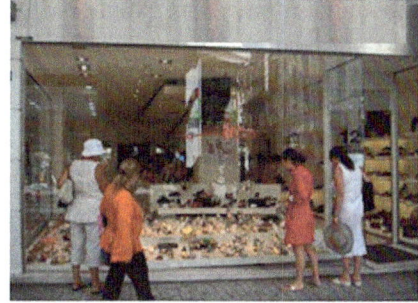

Russian shops - unattributed

Sixty years on and Iron Lung treatment for polio is virtually obsolete, replaced by an idea originally conceived in the 1790's by Edward Jenner who noticed that milk maids who regularly came into contact with cowpox rarely contracted the more virulent smallpox. His brilliant leap of imagination was to wonder what would happen if he infected a young boy with cowpox before exposing him to the smallpox virus.

He did just that and the child did not contract smallpox. Consequently an entire vaccination industry was born and now polio vaccine has been so successful, India had only two cases of polio in 2010. But there is no room for complacency, Polio is making a comeback. According to the World Health Organization in 2012 there was an increase in Nigeria to forty three cases which means it could regain its grip across Africa. So despite extensive efforts polio still clings on and who knows if we don't persevere, the Iron Lung may well make a comeback.

Survival of the fittest Imagination.
How many of us have said..."I thought of that." Depressing when you find out that your idea is now someone else's success. But was it really your idea? According to the U.N (2011) seven billion of us occupy the planet and each individual is fermenting a multiplicity of ideas every hour of every waking day. Is it any wonder that Ecclesiastes 1:9 says, "... there is nothing new under the sun."

For an idea to fight its way into reality it has to surmount a host of barriers including; time, place, finance, social circumstances, etc. In 1990's Russia for example, the quantity of 'ideas' for sale was minimal compared to the USA. The Russians were slowly recovering from the horrors of the Second World War and had little disposable income.

Knowing this, my friend paid for a group of schoolgirls from St Petersburg to travel from Birmingham to Oxford Street for a window shopping expedition. Ever the philanthropist he was really excited about introducing them to this new world. Unfortunately he hadn't planned on them marching briskly past the stores to the bottom of Oxford Street where they stopped to gaze in admiration at the towering height of Centre Point. Window shopping simply didn't apply in their 'poor' economy. If they didn't have the cash to buy, what was the reason for looking?

A situation illustrated by the Russian journalist (page 5.) photographing a 1950's butcher chopping a large side of beef, which due to the gaunt faces of the crowd outside must have been a newsworthy occasion. Contrast this with the picture, taken in the Kremlin, fifty years later, showing a much more affluent society with women shoppers looking casually at shoes which they can afford. Therefore always hang on to your 'ideas' and sow them as you would seeds, when conditions are favourable for growth; unfortunately, however, those conditions are not dependant on finance alone, they are also bound up in the social and moral attitudes of the time.

Imagination victim of prejudice.
Occasionally imagination provides spectacular breakthroughs but no matter how exceptional you are if you don't 'fit in', your ideas have little chance of success.
During the Second World War, Alan Turing a young Cambridge University mathematician helped a team at Bletchley Park break the code of the German 'Enigma' machine and shorten the war effort by an incalculable amount. Their success was based on a brilliant deduction Turing made which would not have occurred without our imagination's unique ability to turn current thinking on its head.
Initially the team had focussed on trying to find the correct code combinations to the Enigma until Turing used one of imaginations unique capabilities... he turned the thought on its head by saying:
"From a contradiction, you can deduce everything."

His reasoning was that as there were many more false code combinations than correct combinations, why waste time trying to find all the correct combinations? Instead start by getting rid of the 'contradictions', first.
In other words don't look for the needle in the haystack get rid of the hay, which will leave the needles exposed.

Imagination - victim of prejudice

In May 940 two 'Turing Bombes', (electronic cryptanalytic machines) called Victory and Aggie started looking for and excluding 'contradictory' combinations and successfully decoded 178 messages, in particular passing on information about the German plans for Dunkirk, which gave the allies enough extra time to evacuate and save untold number of lives.

Of all the leading code breakers at Bletchley, Turing was regarded by many as a genius because he also invented the first ever 'stored-program computer' (stores program instructions in electronic memory). But his computer work, though light years ahead of its time, was ignored because his homosexuality was perceived as a danger to the Country.

Criminally prosecuted in 1952 he was forced to accept chemical castration (treatment with female hormones), as an alternative to prison. Sadly he died in 1954, just two weeks before his 42nd birthday from cyanide poisoning which some say was injected into a half eaten apple they found beside his bed.

Following an Internet campaign in 2009, Prime Minister Gordon Brown made an official public apology for the way he was treated after the war. Even NASA had said that without his ideas their computer development would have been set back many years.

Fittingly 2012 is also 'Alan Turing Year' in recognition of his work and influence. But perhaps his most appropriate epitaph is the statue of him sitting on a bench unveiled in a Manchester park 2011 which bears the inscription 'Father of computer science, mathematician, logician, wartime codebreaker, victim of prejudice'.

Nature is obsolete.
We are part of Nature and Nature exists as a biological entity within a physical world. On the face of it in a no-contest situation. Soft-edge Nature pitted against a hard-edge environment, no chance. It's like matching a caterpillar against a rock.

The rock should far outlast the caterpillar, yet it's the caterpillar that endures due to the most primitive drive of all - to become immortal. Something seemingly impossible for any flesh and blood creature to do, because the physical world keeps battering it with a host of shock waves constantly hammering away with wind, water, extremes of temperature and if that isn't enough, chemical assault from volcanoes.

It's extremely wearing so the only way Nature can become immortal is to keep repairing the damage and when those repair mechanisms eventually wear out, renew herself and start afresh as a new individual.

But now Nature is obsolete. As obsolete as the eighty percent of genes we carry round in our own gene pools today.

For in the year of our Lord 2003 the living world was totally changed, forever. The event was heralded in June 2000 when the International g30 Sequencing Consortium announced the production of a draft of the human genome sequence and then three years later in April, 2003 it produced the completed version of our own genome sequence.

At last we, Homo sapiens, have not only unearthed an instruction manual containing the key building blocks for every human on the planet but we can now read, assemble, and more importantly re-assemble them.

This is probably the most stunning achievement our species is ever likely to accomplish as it paves the way for everything that will surely follow; from possible cures for all genetic illness to the creation of super-beings designed for any function we can imagine, from deep space travellers to super-hero athletes.

We have outstripped Nature and are now the masters of our universe and will decide our own evolutionary development, for good or ill.

All become possible due to this one simple, some say most blessed others most catastrophic, evolutionary event ever... Imagination.

THE BIOLOGICAL JOURNEY

"Imagination not only creates life but prevents it."

R.C-T 2012

Imagination begets Imagination

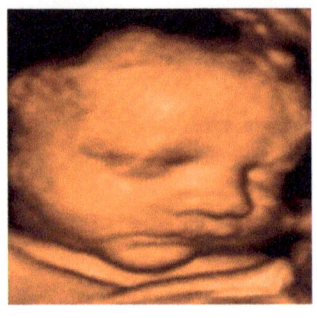

thisismy.co.uk

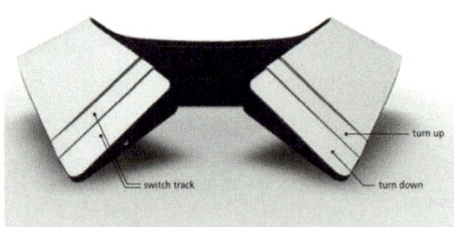

Music for Deaf people Frederik Podzuweit

Homo sapiens' journey to Imagination starts at conception but not in a way we would expect, for although nature has been the driving force behind evolution since the very first life form evolved billions of years ago, in some of our 'civilised societies,' evolutions role has now been demoted to that of an onlooker. Procreation can only succeed with the consent of the living.

Reality is much stranger than fiction and if the rest of the animal kingdom could comprehend the concept of family planning they'd be amazed not only at the way we practice 'life control' but especially the way we so readily extend that courtesy to other species. Dairy cows have no say in the choice of a bull when they are artificially inseminated whilst Zoo animal numbers are controlled without their permission as illustrated by this headline from Sky News in July 2006; "Bonking Big Cats on Birth Control at Bangladesh Zoo."

It's no different in the home where we happily take our domestic pets to be surgically 'neutered', a euphemistic term if ever there was one. Whilst in the USA the Alliance for Contraception in Cats &Dogs aim to humanely control their populations worldwide by non surgical sterilisation mainly by injections of Zinc gluconate.

As usual Imagination is constantly sophisticating techniques and now American pet owners can obtain a twelve month reversible contraception for their 'lady dogs' by means of a silicone implant (hopefully not industrial grade.)
Which perfectly illustrates how Imagination not only creates life but prevents it.

If conception is no longer the excusive property of Nature but also dependent on the vagaries of human Imagination, then it is no different for the development of the human foetus.

In order to progress successfully through its amazing forty week journey from the most primitive stages of life to our current status at the top of the evolutionary ladder, incredible as it may seem, it needs the consent of Imagination. For we have reached a stage in our evolution where neither God nor Nature is the final arbiter in the birth of a human being, Imagination begets Imagination.

The point is best illustrated if we examine the main stages of foetal development in its journey to Imagination. The critical stage occurs at five weeks when the Cerebral Cortex, a feature unique to Homo sapiens, starts to develop and at nine weeks the foetus can bend and react to loud sounds and make avoidance movements in response to being stroked on the cheek with a hair. This sensitivity quickly extends to the genital area (ten weeks), palms (eleven weeks), then soles of the feet (twelve weeks), at which stage it also starts sucking its thumb.

By seventeen weeks all parts of the abdomen and buttocks are sensitive and at thirty two weeks nearly every part of the body reacts to the same hair stroke.

This is all down to our skin, that marvellously complex organ which in every adult contains a hundred varieties of cells per square inch and a thousand nerve endings all especially sensitive to heat, cold, pressure and pain. Skin also respond to noise as researchers in Belfast found when they beamed a 250-500 Hz pulse of sound at a sixteen week old foetus and noted a clear behavioural response (Shahidullah and Hepper, 1992). This was surprising as 'ears' don't become functional for another eight weeks. What was especially significant is that 'reactive listening' begins before 'hearing'. Indicating that in primal human development hearing began through the skin and skeletal framework, long before we used ears as our primary organ for listening.

Clearly a major information channel it is possible that it inspired German designer Frederik Podzuweit (previous page) to invent a lightweight collar which converts music through a vibrating membrane, transmitting sound via the neck and shoulders to the temporal lobe. I mention this invention as it perfectly illustrates H. sapiens unique ability to associate facts and theory together with a perceived need, 'prior' to finding a successful solution.

At week ten the foetus is in control of stretching its arms and practicing breathing by inhaling and exhaling amniotic fluid.

Cerebral v Biological

Between eleven to fifteen weeks a sense of smell and taste develops in response to chemicals in the amniotic fluid and by fourteen weeks swallowing increases with sweet tastes and decreases with sour.
By fifteen weeks its taste buds already look like a mature adult's and doctors know that the amniotic fluid can smell strongly of curry and other spices from a mother's diet.

At sixteen weeks foetus have been known to react to AFT (amniotic fluid test) - a procedure in which a small amount of amniotic fluid containing foetal tissue is extracted for testing for chromosomal abnormalities and foetal infections. Their heart rates may oscillate, they may shrink away from the needle, or they may turn and attack it if it catches them. Others remain motionless and their breathing may not return to normal for several days, which can be upsetting for both parents and doctors watching the foetus's responses via ultrasound.

The evidence also proved upsetting to others as well. In 2008 proponents sought to pass a bill reducing the limit for abortions to 20 weeks which was supported by David Cameron now the Tory leader.

Gordon Brown the then Prime Minister and a majority of MPs voted to keep the current limit of 24 weeks, so the bill was defeated making abortion legal in England and Wales at 24 weeks if two doctors agree to one of the following; having a baby would upset your mental or physical health more than having an abortion; having the baby would harm the mental or physical health of any children you already have.

In June 2010 a report commissioned by the Department of Health from the Royal College of Obstetricians and Gynaecologists stated that nerve endings in the brain of a foetus are not sufficiently formed to enable pain to be felt before 24 weeks. So it was their opinion the foetus cannot experience pain in any way prior to this period.

Professor Allan Templeton, president of the Royal College who chaired the review, said that the research put forward by anti-abortion campaigners that a human foetus did in fact feel pain at or before 24 weeks was based on evidence from premature babies and did not apply to the foetus in the womb.

A second finding stated that the foetus is naturally sedated and unconscious in the womb leading the panel to advice that anaesthetics for the foetus are not needed when it is terminated.

Voluntary termination!

However, Ultrasound pioneer, Professor Stuart Campbell, from London's King's College Hospital, disagreed. His view was that while he was in favour of women having choice, he thought the limit should be reduced to 20 weeks saying:

"To me it is almost barbaric to abort foetuses between 20 and 24 weeks... between 20 to 24 weeks the foetus is really quite advanced in terms of its nervous system. It has facial expressions, it can open its eyelids, it will react to a needle being put on its skin." And Professor Campbell, who co-incidentally produced scans in 2004 of a 12-week-old foetus apparently 'womb-walking', added: "It is developing in such a way that it deserves to keep its hold on life."

Whatever the arguments it is estimated that there are 200,000 legal abortions performed annually in the U.K. and according to the Mail Online (May 2008), in Europe more than one in five pregnancies are terminated each year. Recently the whole question of the legal basis for a termination was again thrown into the spotlight when the Department of Health (February 2012), launched an investigation into the secret filming of doctors at British clinics allegedly admitting they were prepared to falsify paperwork to arrange illegal abortions, based on sex-selection. In October 2012 Government Health Secretary, Jeremy Hunt, announced that he would favour a change in the law to halve the limit on abortions from 24 weeks to 12 weeks.

Homo sapiens' cerebral dominion over Nature's biological domain.
Critics say this is too early, as testing for genetic defects is not currently viable at 12 weeks. But at least the debate has started in earnest and hopefully it will bring into sharp relief the issues surrounding the exact criteria required to terminate a foetus, which will lead onto an even wider moral debate i.e. at what stage do terminations become Eugenics?

Having followed albeit briefly the amazing developmental journey of the human foetus, you will have your own view. My purpose has been to use this debate as a prime example of Homo sapiens' cerebral dominion over Nature's biological domain and the power that the dominant 'Ideology (imagination), of a society has over life and death. A feature unparalleled in the animal kingdom as no other species undergoes voluntary termination!

THE NIGHTMARE OF SLEEP

Every night we are rendered unconsciousness
by an unknown assailant.

R.C-T 2012

The unknown assailant

Our search for Imagination will continue through the development of the human foetus but it is now time for us to undertake a daytime journey through the realms of Sleep. However I must warn you it is not for the fainthearted, as I guarantee that on your return you will never commit your head to a pillow in quite the same way again. Every night we lose grip on our precious reality, for no matter how hard we rub our eyes sleep will get us in the end.

Incredible, probably the most advanced species in the universe is rendered unconscious every night by an unknown assailant and although we can walk on the moon and design the most sophisticated weaponry and computers ...we can still do nothing about it. Not surprising therefore, that since the dawn of man dream interpretation has been big business.

The Romans believed that dreams made predictions about the future and Aristotle thought dreams could diagnose illness. Egyptians credited 'dream interpreters' as having a divine gift, whilst North American Indians welcome dreaming as a channel by which their ancestors communicate with them. Others are more apprehensive, some Chinese believe their souls leave the body to enter the dream world and if they wake suddenly they are in danger of leaving it there, leading to a deep mistrust of alarm clocks in case they go off by accident.

Predictably Medieval society tried to control dreaming by condemning it; Benedict Peterius, a Jesuit priest: said "The devil is most always implicated in dreams, filling the minds of men with poisonous superstition and not only uselessly deluding but perniciously deceiving them." After that only a fool would dare confess to dreaming.
Imagine their fate if anyone had admitted to have dreamt that in the 21st century people would put dirty dishes in a box at night and bring them out clean in the morning!

The early 19th century was more pragmatic, simply dismissing dreams as the result of external noises, indigestion or anxiety until the end of that century when Sigmund Freud, explained dreaming as the 'royal road to the unconscious', where the subconscious shaped dreams as wish-fulfilment. Freud's theories have slipped into obscurity but he may well have been near the truth as we will discuss later.
Certainly Shakespeare's line "To sleep perchance to dream," was scientifically justified in 1947 when the American EEG (graphical record of electrical brain activity) Society, was founded to start serious research into the phenomena of Sleep.

Making sense out of nonsense
Activation synthesis theory .
The first and critical observation came in 1953 when Aserinsky and Kleitman described REM sleep at the Society's inauguratory International congress. Their breakthrough research found that at certain periods during the night peoples eyeballs started moving erratically under their lids and more importantly if woken they reported experiencing vivid dreams.

The link was made, REM (Rapid Eyeball Movement) during sleep equals dreaming. Unfortunately their early research did not tell the full story. It only explained one aspect of sleep and because every living person on the planet can identify with dreaming their results became interpreted as the principal reason for sleep i.e. we are tired and need to physically rest and in doing so we dream. In other words the principal reason for sleeping is to relieve muscle fatigue. Nothing could be further from the truth and it was not until the sixties that scientists discovered to their astonishment that sleep not only consisted of an extra four completely different stages but what was really unbelievable was that during REM sleep we lose all control of our body's skeletal muscles i.e we are rendered totally immobile!
Yet the importance of 'dreaming' had become so embedded in the scientific communities' psyche that little credence was given to any of these findings. The only thing it did was to offer a scientific explanation for the terrifying experience of waking during the night to find you can't move a muscle, by explaining that it was a physiological occurrence rather than a ghost, or goblin, sitting on your chest, which had been embedded in folk-lore for centuries. So it was quietly assumed that sleep paralysis was simply nature's way of preventing you from acting out your dreams and left at that.

Unfortunately the inference although so near, was so far from the truth ,that it would obscure the real truth for at least another decade. Until December 1977, when John Allan Hobson and Robert McCauley set the cat amongst the pigeons when they published their 'Activation synthesis theory' in the American Journal of Psychiatry. Having studied the differences in neuronal activity of the brainstem during waking and REM sleep they noticed that REM sleep was accompanied by the random firing of neurons in the cerebral cortex. For the first time their observations offered a different reason for the bizarre unconscious state we call dreaming by proposing that dreaming was simply a result of our forebrain attempting to make 'sense out of nonsense'. Yet such is the power of cognitive dissonance (the psychological discomfort caused by trying to hold opposing facts) that Scientists tried to reduce their discomfort by admitting that although dreams often made no sense, the subjects eyes were still watching a film but it was a surreal film such as L'Age d'Or by Luis Buñuel and Salvador Dalí.

In other words rapid eyeball movement still meant the eyes were watching a film and that dreaming was the prime reason for sleeping, but again though near the truth they were still far away from the real truth.

Hobson and McCauley's research raised important questions, i.e. If dreaming is simply the result of our brains trying to make sense out of nonsense then why do we have to be knocked unconscious whilst were sleeping? Why would the brain shut down our skeletal muscle control to stop us physically acting out 'random' thoughts yet leave our eyes free to watch?
To find the answers, which are even more incredible than the questions, it will help if we start by considering the development of sight in the human foetus.
At the beginning of the twenty first century scientists discovered that premature infants can see light and shape (Eswaran et al., 2002), so it was generally assumed that a foetus could see in the womb. This appeared to confirm earlier findings by Japanese scientists who reported a physical reaction to flashes of light shone at a 24 week old premature infant. In the same year Curtis Lowery and colleagues from the University of Arkansas used a non invasive technique MEG (magnetoencephalography), to record brain responses from a foetus exposed to a light flashed intermittently over its mother's abdomen for a six-minute period. But out of ten foetuses aged between 28wks and 36wks, only four showed some sort of brain response. As only 40% of the subjects showed any brain activity and all were a lot older in developmental terms than the Japanese infant it is reasonable to assume that 'sight' had no part to play in the Japanese findings .
No explanation has been offered as yet for this discrepancy between these two findings but as the skin is such a fantastically sensitive organ perhaps the foetal skin was sensing the light rays just as it had in 'reactive listening'. However it is important in establishing a time line for the development of sight as previously, in 1981, J.C. Birnholz had already discovered that a 23wk sleeping foetus experiences REM sleep in the same way an adult does. This suggests that at twenty three weeks a foetus is experiencing dreaming even though its brain is not wired up to process visual signals. Which casts doubt on the original theory that REM sleep equals 'visual dreaming', in other words what are foetal dreams about if they're not visual and what events are the eyes watching if they can't see?
Surely this was the first clue to suggest that eye movement was simply a by-product of a particular stage of sleep?
Or are we now to believe that that we are rendered immobile every night to experience dreaming which apparently has nothing to do with vision? Curiouser and curiouser!

Sleep does not suddenly evolve from a resting brain

After fifty years of research William Dement, co-founder of Stanford University's Sleep Research Centre was quoted in the May 2010 edition of National Geographic as saying. "As far as I know, the only reason we need to sleep that is really, really solid is because we get sleepy."
True enough, but he didn't explain why we get sleepy.

Fortunately the reason had already been published one year earlier in 2009 when Mathematician Karin Schwab and a team of neuroscientists at Friedrich Schiller University in Jena, put forward what proved to be an explosive new theory.

Experimenting on a fifteen week old sheep foetus, which has a similar type of brain development to ours, they recorded electrical brain activity which indicated that it entered a sleep-like state weeks before any rapid eye movements were detected.

Conceding that it was difficult to imagine what an immature foetus experienced during such cycles the researchers came to the conclusion that their results shed new light on the origins of sleep by established that;

"Sleep does not suddenly evolve from a resting brain. Sleep and sleep state changes are active regulated processes."

Just like breathing (no matter how long you try to hold your breath you will be forced to gulp in air eventually), sleep is beyond our conscious control. We don't fall asleep because we feel physically or mentally tired, we sleep when our body makes us.

Karin Schwab's finding were huge, for the first time in our evolutionary history she had unmasked the Sandman. Our own body is the culprit, we knock ourselves out every night!

A finding incredible enough in itself but what is even more incredible is that the serious implications haven't filtered through to the top echelons of society, let alone the public, because the cause of sleep is almost universally misunderstood. We still think that falling asleep in the wrong social setting is joke, a social faux pas, or a deliberate slight. Witness the audiences who laugh at 'old men', dropping off in the middle of a comedy sketch not realising the seriousness of the real life implications.

Sure sleep can be facilitated i.e. settling down for a nap after a meal makes sense as you would not be able to undertake physical activity, but the fact that we don't understand that sleep is beyond any form of conscious control is evidenced by the sad but ironic fate of the aforementioned pioneer of sleep research, Eugene Aserinsky

He died in a car accident in July 1998 after falling asleep at the wheel, he was seventy seven.

But Aserinsky's was not an isolated case; unfortunately it's a worldwide phenomenon. In 2009 the USA National Highway Traffic Safety Administration estimated that the euphemism 'drowsy driving', results in 1,550 deaths, 71,000 injuries and more than 100,000 accidents each year in that country alone.

In the UK driver 'fatigue'(a misnomer if ever there was one, because if it is physical fatigue, you can simply get out and stretch your legs), is responsible for 20% of traffic accidents on long journeys, particularly motorways.

Yet it is not older men but those under thirty who are more likely to have a sleep related vehicle accident. Also considering our bodies are programmed to sleep at night, it comes as no surprise that the greatest risk of falling asleep at the wheel is between midnight and 6am.

But sleep accidents are not restricted to motorways it affects all other methods of transport including ships, trains and planes, and what's worse it's worldwide.

Charles Lindbergh perfectly captures the effects of sleep when he describes his 1927 transatlantic flight:
"My mind clicks on and off. I try letting one eyelid close at a time while I prop the other with my will. But the effect is too much, sleep is winning, my whole body argues dully that nothing, nothing life can attain is quite so desirable as sleep. My mind is losing resolution and control."

To counteract the Lindbergh effect pilots have traditionally been allowed to work in pairs, so one can whilst the other stays alert, but even this is no safeguard. The insidious nature of sleep infiltrates even air-flight support staff. In October 2007, UK Airport News Info reported that four air traffic controllers had been suspended at an Italian airport after it emerged they had been sleeping while on duty. In February 2008, a 'Go.' airline flight overshot the airport in Hawaii by approximately thirty miles before circling back over the sea. Having originally said they had entered the wrong air-traffic-control frequency both pilots later admitted they had fallen asleep.

In May 2010, BBC NEWS reported that a dozing pilot was to blame for a plane crash in southern India which killed 158 people. Although an official investigation report had not been released, the Hindustan Times said that data recorders captured the sound of snoring leading some people to argue that perhaps it is time pilots left their microphones on permanently.

"Physician, heal thyself"

But these events do not seem to have raised alarm bells with the aviation authorities.

Early in 2012, the House of Commons Transport Committee heard evidence from the British Airline Pilots Association (BALPA) warning that even more passengers' lives will be put at risk due to new EU rules which would allow pilots to fly as far as California without back-up crew; work up to seven early starts in a row, and land their aircraft after 22 hours without sleep.

Despite the above evidence the Civil Aviation Authority rejected any suggestion that the controversial EU rules would compromise safety (I presume their safety not ours!).

The argument continues but one wonders if the C.A.A. understands that sleep is an actively regulated process? You can't blame them if they don't; as it wasn't until August 2009 that junior doctors, in the UK, had their working hours officially reduced from 100 hours a week to 48 hours a week. And the fact still hasn't got through to Doctors' organisations who criticised the European Working Time Directive, saying the reduced hours means there is too little time to provide training. May be so but there are no records as to how many patients health were put at risk by junior doctors falling asleep prior to 2009. There is plenty of allegorical evidence though; take for example the case of the junior doctor who, tired as he was, desperately wanted to sit with a terminally ill patient and be with them in their last moments. Sitting beside her he took hold of her hand, and much to his dismay awoke to find he had fallen asleep at the critical moment. Methinks this proverb from Luke 4:23, is appropriate "Physician, heal thyself".

The land of sleep is a perilous place, because up till now we have not understood the real reason for its existence or function. But sleep holds the key to discovering the biological nature of Imagination,so it is time to start unravelling its mysteries and the first step will be to examine the minute electrical discharges we call brainwaves.

* the curtain of sleep does not fall every eighteen hours, if differs from individual to individual as presumably we can delay sleeps onset , to a certain extent, for self-preservation reasons .

* Randy Gardner holds the world record for staying awake (Wikipedia). He lasted eleven days before sleep got him but experienced poor concentration, short term memory, paranoia, and hallucinations. Many other claim to have stayed awake for longer but they have not been scientifically observed ,as many individuals think they are awake but are in reality experience multi periods of Micro Sleep.

THIS IS YOUR BRAIN SPEAKING

"It's one of the biggest mysteries of cognition, what controls your thoughts".

Medindia Health News 2012-11-25

Electrical activity generated by the brain.

According to the National Academy of Sciences, "A human brain has a greater number of possible connections among its nerve cells than the total number of atomic particles in the universe."

I doubt Dr Hans Berger knew of the statistics, back in 1924, when he invented the electroencephalograph (EEG) and produced the first recording of electrical activity generated by the brain. For it now appears that it is the minute electrical charge generated by billions of neurons connecting with each other that causes an electrical wave which can be detected by electrodes on the scalp. Berger was very cautious about his results and as it turned out he had every right to be because, when he published them five years later, they were met with incredulity and derision by the German medical and scientific establishment.

Perhaps his results were too close to Frankenstein fiction but eventually history authenticated his work and now scientists divide brainwaves into four main categories Beta; Alpha; Theta and Delta. It seems hard to believe that the incredible complexity of our cognitive functions depend on only four types of brainwave .
Yet it is the synthesis of these tiny, almost insignificant, electrical discharges that not only make us uniquely human but perhaps more important, a unique human being.

Although Berger's pioneering work was initially ridiculed it paved the way for the announcement nearly ninety years later that researchers could actually understand our thoughts. In January 2012, Neuroscientists at the University of California, Berkeley, experimented with recording the brain activity of subjects whilst they listened to a series of spoken words. When they ran the data back through a computer programme the self same words were repeated through their processors speakers.

The work may have been triggered back in 2009 when the USA Army Research Office donated $4 million to the University of California, Irvine, to try and identify imagined speech so that soldiers during combat could connect telepathically with each other using a hand held computer. They say nothing good comes out of war but these results have the potential for helping people such as Professor Stephen Hawking, and others with locked-in syndrome, to communicate their thoughts to the outside world and currently a team headed by neuroscientist Philip Low, at NeuroVigil, of San Diego have invented the 'iBrain', a headband without countless external electrodes, which allows communication outside the lab.

Types of Brain Waves

Although the technology to enable 'thinking aloud' has come of age, it is only used during our conscious states and as yet has revealed little about the functions of brain waves during sleep.

Brainwaves are ultra-low frequency electromagnetic waves emitting such minute electrical discharges they wouldn't light a single LED, yet they are responsible for the functioning of all complex life on Earth. They are so critical to our understating of the biological basis of Imagination that it is crucial to examine their role in closer detail.

TYPES OF BRAIN WAVES.

Our brains generate six types of brainwave in total, of which three are exclusive to sleep. They all have their own distinct signature and wave formation which not only varies in voltage, height and depth but the number of times each waves peaks in a second.

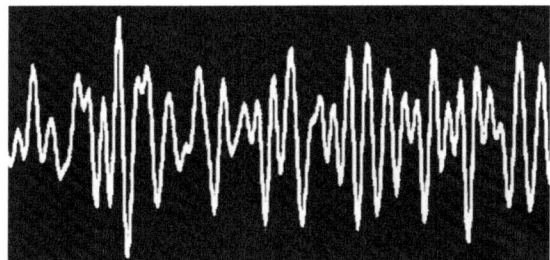

14 - 30+ Hz. per second
BETA waves - lowest voltage and highest frequency.
Our waking periods are defined by unpredictability and although each moment may be similar, it is never exactly the same as the one before. Which means the brain has to continually process,store and evaluate incoming information by comparing it to existing memories so it can give instructions as to how to proceed.

Beta waves are generated both when were awake and asleep (more later) and are are always in a state of flux which means they are 'desynchronous' i.e. they don't have any consistent pattern . Their output has been measured from fourteen waves per second(14Hz) to a massive eighty waves(- 80Hz). This is because Beta waves generation increases in direct response to the complexity of a task e.g. from reading a book to playing sport.

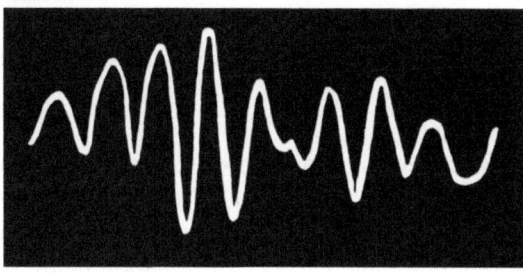

9-14 Hz. per second
ALPHA waves

Alpha waves are wider and slower than Beta waves with higher peaks and lower troughs and occur at a lesser frequency, from 9Hz to 14 Hz. They are produced when were in 'chill' mode and significantly are generated whenever we are 'thinking , especially when we close our eyes or relax.

As you sit unwinding for the day with shoes off ,and perhaps a refreshing drink, Alpha waves start mixing with Beta waves, dampening down there activity to produce a gentle state of 'reverie' which some say is similar to that experienced by people who smoke marijuana or drink alcohol. Interestingly long term regular marijuana users show an increase in alpha wave production even when they have refrained from use for 24 hours. But more important they also occur in Slow wave sleep which we will discuss later.

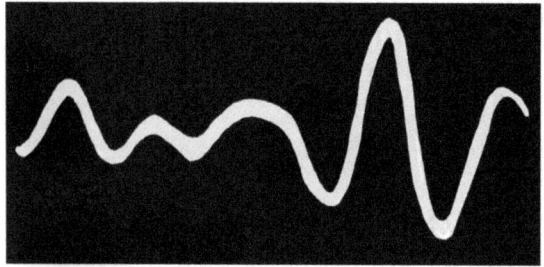

4-8 Hz. per second
THETA waves

Theta waves are slower again than Alpha waves (between 4Hz and 8Hz), and are generated as your attention to new tasks becomes minimal. Typically experienced by drivers on motorways who get those 'good ideas' yet can't remember if they have passed the last service station. The problem is that as Theta waves start to predominate over Alpha waves it means your body is preparing you for the descent into deep sleep, which is a dangerous situation to be in at 70 miles per hour. So for the reasons already discussed take a break from driving as soon as possible, have a nap if necessary (see the importance of sleep spindles later), until your brain kicks back into Beta mode to cope with complexities of driving.

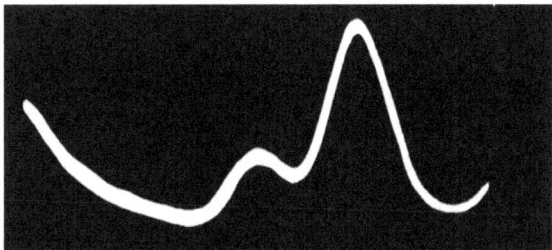

0.1-3.0 Hz. per second
DELTA waves (Highest voltage- lowest frequency

Delta waves occur when you are asleep or in a coma, and are the slowest of all brain waves ranging from only a tenth of a cycle up to three cycles per second. They are so slow you are, to all intents and purposes, 'dead to the world' which means the brain can get on with directing the bodies core maintenance work and more important, for our purposes its psychological ,maintenance. Delta waves may be slow but their high voltage reflects the intensity of the work they do.

Deep sleep is so effective in 'body repair' that Doctors often follow natures practice and keep patients in a medically induced coma to give the body chance to repair itself. Distressing as it may appear to those visiting loved ones in Intensive Care, once they realise its purpose it can go a long way to easing their distress. The hard part is understanding that the patient has no concept of time and that getting better can take an excruciatingly long time ... for the relatives.

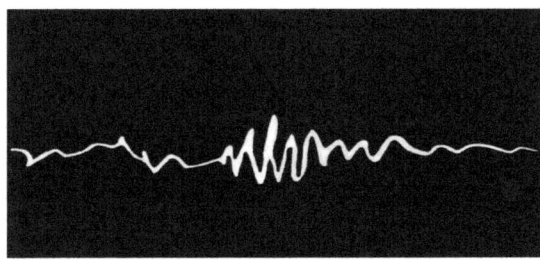

Vary in speed per second
SLEEP SPINDLES

Sleep spindles only occur as your body temperature drops and your heart rate slows as you drift into sleep. Previously there had been little explanation as to their function even though they are generated for almost fifty percent of the total sleep cycle i.e. nearly four hours every night.

The illustration above shows that although they don't have the same amplitude they are frequent and desynchronous (i.e. random), which would indicate they are busy processing something.

Sleep Spindles

Trouble was nobody knew what was being processed until earlyIn 2011 when a study led by Matthew Walker, associate professor of psychology and neuroscience at the University of California, Berkeley, discovered that sleep spindles act as carriers of information.

This was the crucial piece of the jigsaw which helped eventually solve the question;"What happens to incredible amount of information we manage to absorb during our sixteen hour waking day, every day, for the whole of our lives, and just as important how is it stored and sorted into useful memories and junk memories?"It had been known for some time that all our waking experiences are stored as memories in the hippocampus and the hippocampus has a limited storage capacity, i.e. once it's full it's full. Which means if it can't empty itself to allow for the storage of new memories then like any 'full' memory card a message would say, "sorry not enough memory space" and we would be stuck forever in the past, reliant on old memories.

Walker and co's research initially pointed to sleep being the regulator of our daily memories based on the (some would say obvious) fact, that individuals who experienced a full eight hours sleep felt more refreshed when they woke and their capacity for learning and memorizing facts improved considerably afterwards. On the face of it this may seem obvious and of little significance but what is significant is what happened when they tested a group of over forty young adults.

In the day, the full group were subjected to a series of demanding memory tests deliberately intended to clog up the hippocampus. When they were examined, afterwards, all the subjects performed to a similar standard. Then the group was divided into two, one half slept for 90 minutes while the others stayed awake. That evening, the two halves joined together and were subjected to another session of learning. When the group was tested directly after this session, they found that the ability to remember the new information deteriorated for those who had remained awake but those who had slept during the day scored higher. In other words their ability to remember had considerably improved because by sleeping in the day they had emptied the information stored in their hippocampus, and could therefore remember new information.

The results (confirmed by EEG measurements,) showed a direct correlation between the amount of sleep spindles produced by each individual in the sleeping group and their ability to absorb new knowledge. This was supported by further evidence which linked activity between sleep spindles, and two areas critical to memory i.e. the hippocampus and prefrontal cortex, (the word 'memories' is used in the broadest sense as everything we experience is stored as a memory, even the most trivial sensation.)

Strategy when studying for exams

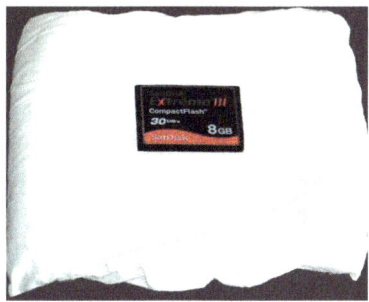

Memory card on pillow.

The Berkley study indicated that sleep spindles, generated in the thalamus, empty the hippocampus of its memories by transferring them to the prefrontal cortex, leaving the hippocampus empty and ready to store new learning experiences. In our eco conscious world it is certainly is an efficient recycling process using exactly the same method we use to free up memory on a flash card i.e. by uploading its photo's directly onto your hard drive. Which means you can use the flash card again and again. The only difference is that our biological 'uploading' is *actioned* by sleep spindles so it only works when an individual is asleep. The Berkeley findings are important as it begins to explain why short term memory is limited and varies from individual to individual, possibly due to the different storage capacity of their hippocampus or how long they have slept for.

It also provide a reason for the tendency to get muddled and find difficulty in remembering new information the longer we go without sleep, simply because the hippocampus is full and cannot store any new information. As an aside the Berkley study also provides a new strategy for anyone studying for exams. Historically students have adopted the 'burn the candle' approach, by staying up studying till the early hours, to arrive, bleary eyed, for the exam the next day. Which doesn't conform to Matthew Walker's discovery "...that we not only need sleep after learning to consolidate what we've memorized, but that we also need it before learning, so that we can recharge and soak up new information the next day." His evidence suggests that it is much more effective to take an exam after a good night's sleep (gives the brain a chance to transfer all the information stored in the hypothalamus), as well as to start studying after a good night's sleep (as the hypothalamus is empty), then take another short sleep, 'between' studies, so that sleep spindles can transfer any 'recent learning' to your forebrain, leaving your hippocampus empty and ready to store more information. Doubtless this will depend on circumstances and practicality, but worth considering, nevertheless.

The research points the way but still leaves many unanswered questions e.g."Which memories are transferred first i.e. those studied after or before sleep? As this research is only in its infancy it may well be useful to test it out yourself to see if taking a 'sleep' helps and to what extent? One thing looks certain; make sure you get the full eight hours sleep in, before the exam, so the sleep spindles and REM segments, can complete their work.

Mathew Walker also gives us the first indication as to why we need sleep, he says; "Our findings demonstrate that sleep may selectively seek out and operate on our memory systems to restore their critical functions."

In other words they empty the memory bin so it can store new memories, which further supports Karin Schwab's assertion that sleep is an automatic process regulated by a biological need that is beyond our control.

If you think about it, although our cognitive mechanisms appear extremely sophisticated, there is nothing sophisticated about emptying a bucket full of memories, you simply need to take the time out to do it.

Even then we undoubtedly forget things as even our relatively large forebrains can't store every memory forever, unless you are Kim Peek, the real Rain Man, who memorised the entire content of over twelve thousand books, including the bible. But his attribute also acted as his impairment as he had difficulty coping with life and needed the assistance of his carer. Unfortunately he passed away in December 2009 aged 58, which was sad as, because as far as I am aware, no studies were conducted on his sleep processes to see if they were any differences between him and us mere mortals.**n.b.** Walkers findings also seem to confirm the old adage that if you wish to write an essay. Leave it till the day after learning, as sleep will have put it into a logical order, ready for when you wake (which hopefully will be borne out later in our discussion on the role of Alpha waves).

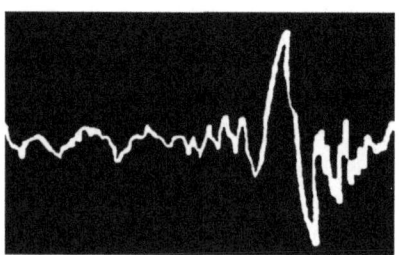 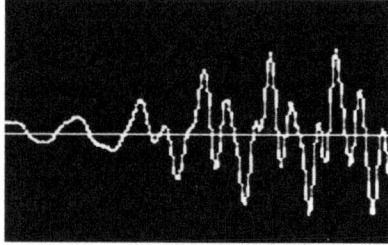

K-Complex   **Sound wave**

If you have ever tried camping out in a tent on a windy night you will understand how difficult it is to get to sleep without ear plugs, yet sleep is such a critical part of living that (as we shall see later), for any animal unfortunate enough to be deprived of it means certain death .

The real purpose of sleep

So it is no accident that Nature devised a method to prevent animals from waking by using the equivalent of 'white noise'(K-complexes), to jam the transmission of external sounds to the brain's auditory regions. This allows the sleep spindles to continue working without interruption as they carry information between the other sleep states. As the sleep spindles increase in duration K-complexes also build in density, increasingly insulating you from any interruption from the outside world. So that you gently progress through slow wave sleep into the 'deepest' segment of slow wave sleep (Delta sleep), where you are virtually unwakeable and often described as 'sleeping like a log'. Having discovered one step in the memory consolidation process i.e. that sleep spindles act as information carriers, we now need to discover what happens to the information they carry.

The real purpose of sleep.
From the foregoing it is clear that there is a lot more to sleep than dreaming yet even when scientists discovered that a night's sleep consisted of another three distinct stages, separate from REM, they confusingly pre-fixed each newly discovered phase with the letter N to stand for Non-REM sleep.
Presumably these phases were seen as secondary and labelled N1; N2; N3 as if they were "Not-Important". Which as it turns out could be nothing further from the truth because, even in this the 21st century, the 'Hollywood' factor surrounding dreaming as the main reason for sleeping is so pervasive that sleep's true purpose is little understood.
So I think it worth examining how each phase interacts with another to see if we can discover, the true purpose of sleep?
The chart on page 31. is worth spending some time on as it shows how each segment of the sleep cycle occurs within a regulated framework and this same framework occurs in every (normal sleeping), human on the planet... every night.

The cycle begins with Stage N1 where Alpha waves are gradually replaced by slower Theta waves which prepare you for stage N2 - the generation of sleep spindles and K-complexes.

N2 blends into N3a when slow Delta waves start to build into Slow wave sleep and as they increase to over 50% we sink into N3b the deepest stage of sleep - Deep sleep.

After a period in Deep sleep the Delta waves decrease as sleep spindles and K-complexes take over followed by a period of REM sleep.
Over eight hours the cycle repeats itself with a slight variation till the last segment of REM, when we move into N1 (Theta) and then wake up.

THE SLEEP CYCLE

How long will you lie there, you sluggard? When will you get up from your sleep?

(Proverbs 6:9)

The sleep cycle framework

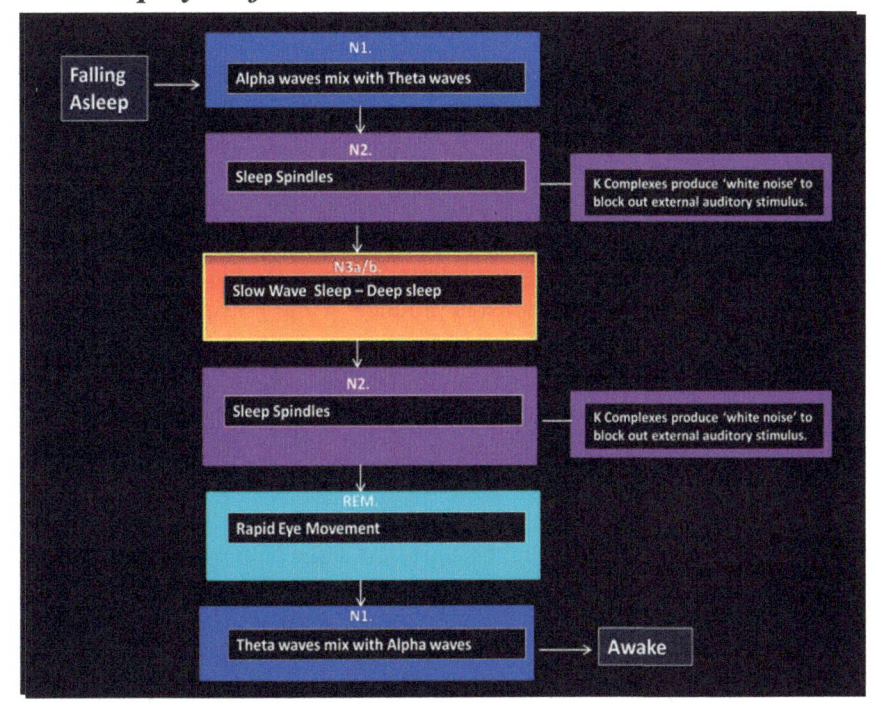

Falling Asleep →

N1. Alpha waves mix with Theta waves
↓
N2. Sleep Spindles — K Complexes produce 'white noise' to block out external auditory stimulus.
↓
N3a/b. Slow Wave Sleep – Deep sleep
↓
N2. Sleep Spindles — K Complexes produce 'white noise' to block out external auditory stimulus.
↓
REM. Rapid Eye Movement
↓
N1. Theta waves mix with Alpha waves → Awake

STAGES OF SLEEP

As we review each separate sleep-stage you will note that a pattern emerges which illustrates not only the sophistication of the process but also shows how each stage is interdependent on another. Which is why going without sleep impairs cognitive performance.

Even marginally interrupting sleep, e.g.going to the toilet,will mean you have trouble getting back into the exact same part of the cycle and may still have to sleep later on to complete the process.

Stage N1. THETA
1-7 mins segments:
Drowsy stage; from Alpha to Theta waves:
Beta waves are gradually replaced by slower Alpha waves which in turn are reduced in frequency until they become Theta waves.

Theta Wave's function is not yet completely understood but they are evidenced by slow rolling eye movements which indicate the brain is no longer reacting to visual information.

There is a loss of some muscle tone and a gradual lack of awareness of your surroundings. However you can still wake with a jerk and some people do, denying they have been asleep.

What is of primary significance, to our discussions later, is that people often report drifting into fantasies or experiencing vague or even vivid hallucinations during Theta, which we need to note contains Alpha waves.

Stage N2. SLEEP SPINDLES
10 - 25 mins segments:

As already described sleep spindles are the information carriers ferrying information between the hypothalamus to Slow wave sleep then Deep sleep and eventually REM. K-complexes produce 'white noise' to help prevent the sleeper waking whilst the sleep spindles are working

Stage N3a & N3b. SLOW WAVE SLEEP to DEEP SLEEP
20- 40 mins segments

High voltage Delta waves occur in all mammals and are a critical part of the sleep process. They occur in two phases; N3a.where Delta wave production is between 20 and 50% (light sleep), and stage N3b. when Delta waves exceed 50%, - the so called Deep sleep stage.

Deep sleep is the period when you are at your most vulnerable rendering you comatose and almost impossible to wake, fortunately it only occurs twice each night, within the first three hours of sleeping.

If you deprive yourself of slow-wave sleep i.e. stay up all night, the next session of Delta sleep will be deeper and longer in recompense, which perhaps explains teenagers' sleep patterns at the weekend.

Interestingly bed-wetting; sleep-walking, sleep-talking and night terrors all occur during Deep sleep periods. They are not uncommon and sleep walking has even been used, successfully, as a defence in a number of criminal proceedings.

Most 'sleep walks', are relatively harmless but involve 'illogical' behaviour such as leaving crisp packets in the fridge or putting the cat out and taking the empty milk bottles back in.

Perhaps the most bizarre was the sad case, in 2004, of a woman who apparently had sex with strangers in her sleep. Her behaviour only came to light when her husband found condoms scattered on the floor in the morning. The activity ceased after psychiatric evaluation, as the expert's, convinced that her case was genuine, by the obvious distress of the couple, helped her with counselling.

Night terrors occur during Deep Sleep, normally in children aged between two and six years, who often sit 'bolt upright', breathing fast with eyes wide open, often screaming in panic, they don't always recognize their parents.

Which is logical if (as we discuss later), they are a result of waking directly from a segment of sleep that has no recourse to memories more than a day old. Alarming as they may seem Night terrors are relatively harmless and current advice (always check with a Doctor) is not to wake children but keep them from hurting themselves perhaps by the judicious arrangement of pillows, but it is most important to remember to keep calm and stay with them. Usually children wake up in a cheerful mood without any recall of the event, unlike their parents.

Sleep walking and night terrors only manifest themselves during Deep sleep and are attributed to the brain trying to go directly to the awake state without ascending through the other stages. Thus leaving an individual in no man's land where, unlike REM, the body is mobile but the brain has no rational control and possibly gets locked into repeating a set of behaviours .

As already stated it is important to note how each separate stage is interdependent on another and that missing out on any sleep stage, impairs cognitive performance the next day. *Or as in the case of older men who have to 'get up in the night', fall asleep during the day as their brain needs to complete the memory transfer process.

Most people who claim to have been burgled in the night without hearing a sound can vouch for the fact that it is almost impossible to wake someone during Deep sleep (see Simon overleaf). The only way to counter the problem is to install a burglar alarm.

Alternately go to bed early, as the most vulnerable time spent in deep sleep occurs during the first 3.0 hrs which , hopefully ,is before burglars set out in the evening. Unlike Father Christmas who must only deliver his presents during the first few hours of sleep as no children ever see him! (hint).

****10% of the sighted population make do with less than six hours sleep every night. Nobody knows why, but it would be reasonable to assume that it cannot be due to them having a larger 'memory bin' as presumably it would take longer to empty. Conversely it is possible they have a smaller storage capacity but that would mean that they would need to sleep more frequently to empty their hypothalamus. The obvious answer is that either the sleep spindles (or all of the mechanisms), work faster but as yet, no one has discovered if the reason is due to inherited or social conditions. If scientists find it's a social effect then perhaps they can spread the word as most people I know don't seem to have enough time in the day as it is.*

Paradoxical sleep

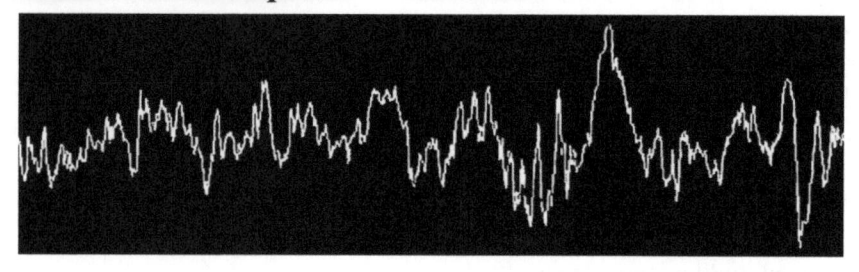

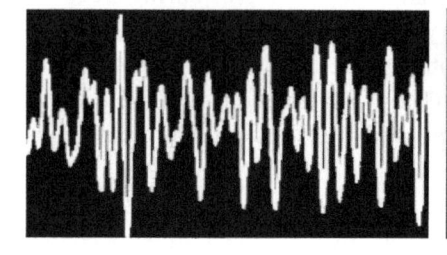

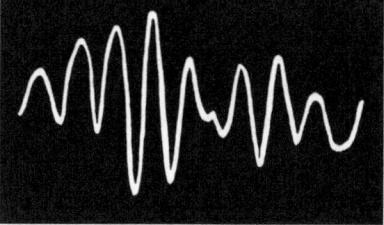

Above REM sleep
Stage 4. REM sleep. 5 - 120 mins.
REM contains both Beta waves (left) and Alpha waves (right).

There are normally five periods of REM sleep during the night. They gradually increase in duration from the first period (between one and seven minutes), to the final period, which lasts for approximately one hour.

This ends abruptly, without sleep spindles, as Theta waves and Alpha waves take over and we wake from the N1 drowsy stage, 'relatively' compos mentis.

The diagram above shows that REM sleep has its own distinctive signature, which is a combination of Alpha and Beta waves (shown separately above)

This indicates that during REM sleep the brain's electrical activity is similar to being awake, except for the one big difference, the body's skeletal muscles are paralyzed. This is why REM sleep is often called 'paradoxical sleep' (self-contradictory) because. your brain is awake but you cannot physically function as if you were awake.

Paradoxical or not, it is worth asking."What is the brain doing during REM periods that merit rendering us immobile?"

Talk about adding insult to injury; not only are our muscles paralysed during each one of the five episodes of REM but the diagram on the next page shows that during the first three hours of the sleep cycle we are also effectively rendered brain-dead on the two occasions when we plunge into Deep sleep ... and this occurs every night of our lives.

Forget horror movies, sleep really is the stuff of nightmares!

Sleeping like a log!

Vulnerability of Deep sleep.

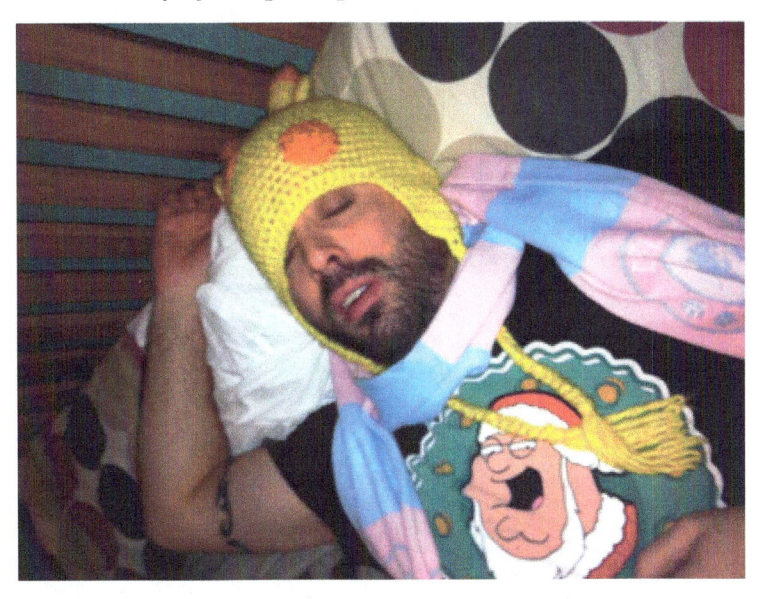

Si, crashed out at a party...

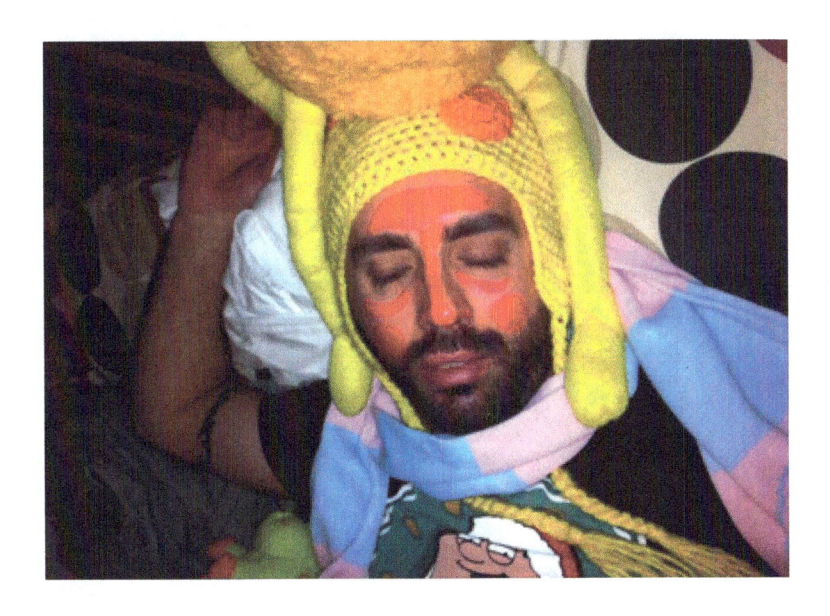

aprox 60 minutes later .

Sleep Cycle Mechanism

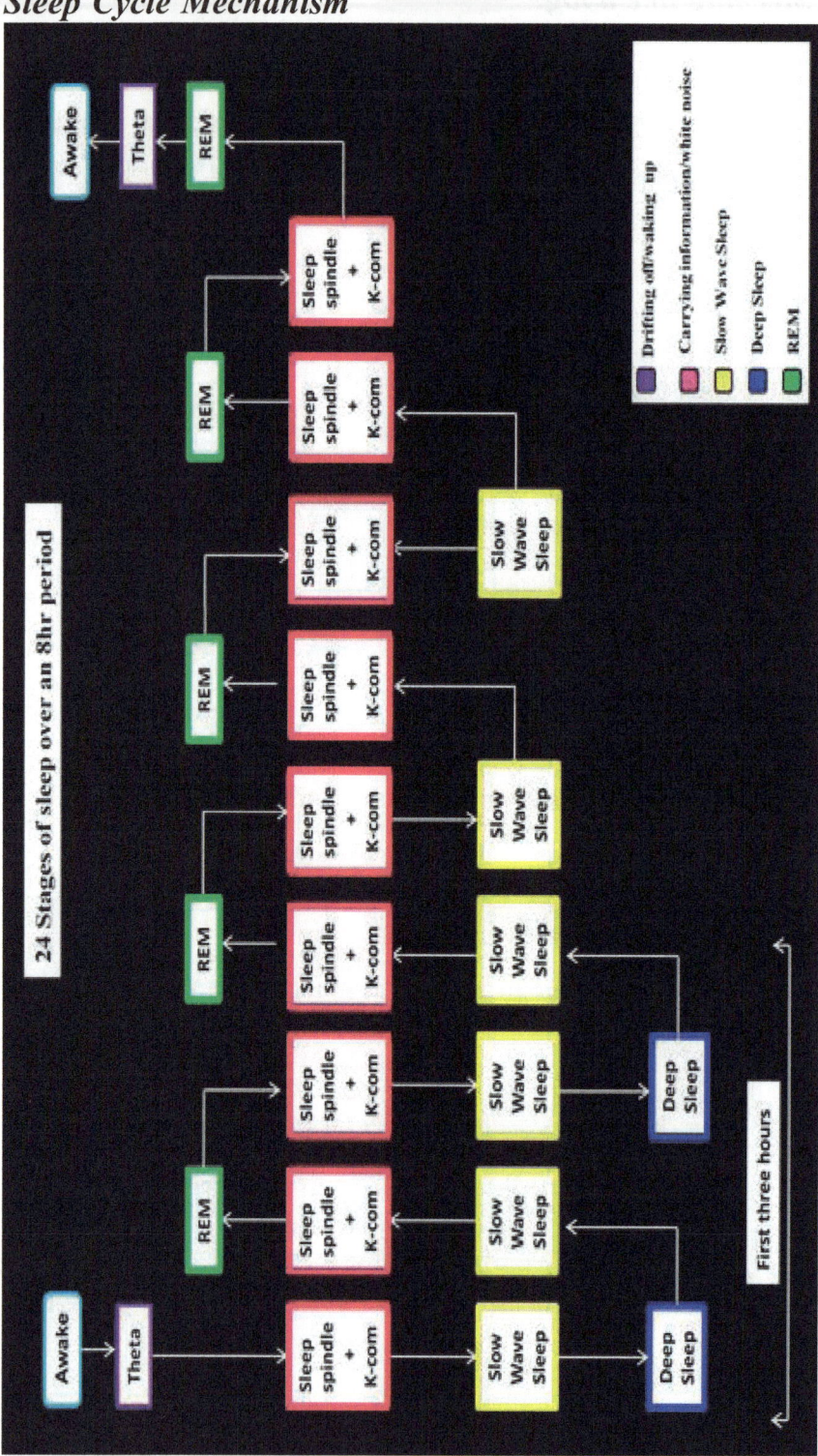

24 Stages of sleep over an 8hr period

Legend:
- ■ Drifting off/waking up
- ■ Carrying information/white noise
- ■ Slow Wave Sleep
- ■ Deep Sleep
- ■ REM

First three hours:

Awake → Theta → Sleep spindle + K-com → Slow Wave Sleep → Deep Sleep

→ Slow Wave Sleep → Sleep spindle + K-com → REM

→ Slow Wave Sleep → Sleep spindle + K-com → Deep Sleep

→ Slow Wave Sleep → Sleep spindle + K-com → REM

→ Slow Wave Sleep → Sleep spindle + K-com → REM

→ Slow Wave Sleep → Sleep spindle + K-com → REM

→ Sleep spindle + K-com → REM

→ Sleep spindle + K-com → REM

→ Theta → Awake

"...and the leopard will lie down with the goat, the calf and the lion and the yearling together."

Isaiah 11:6

REM sleep in animals

Understanding the interdependence of each stage upon the other may well explain some of the psychological effects of sleep disorders where the process is broken or interrupted. If it were possible to re-establish the normal sequence it may also be possible to effect a cure. It may also explain the amnesia experienced by people who recover from a coma induced by trauma, as the brain was plunged into Deep sleep without having chance to generate enough sleep spindles to transfer memories preceding the event, to a REM stage, so they could be saved as long term memories.

This may have important implications for research into memory loss as this form of amnesia may indicate either that the hypothalamus has a finite storage capacity or the retention of new memories is 'time bound' i.e the day's memories may leak away over a period to allow for the storage of newer memories. Whatever the findings it indicates a) how transient memories are and b) how crucial the role of sleep is in organising and permanently recording our memories.

As you trace your finger over the chart on the previous page, you will notice that the sleep cycle follows a regular sequence ; REM plus Slow wave and Deep sleep segments are both followed and preceded by sleep spindles (except for the last REM segment).That they occur in such a formulaic way would suggest that there has to be a critical reason for their structure and especially in their relationship to each other. So it would seem sensible to study each sleep state individually to see if we can gain an understanding of their function. This will enable us to understand how and why they interact with each other in such a specific way. We will start by examining the nature of REM sleep in animals to see if we can trace its evolution in us, Homo imaginus.

REM sleep in animals.
Since the early 1950's, sleep scientist have investigated sleep in virtually every living creature and found that sleep must have evolved at an early stage in our evolution as sleep states are common to amphibians, fish, birds and land mammals. Even the most primitive of organisms such as C. Elegans (a nematode) become lethargic for short periods before each moult and Drosophila (fruit flies,) have been shown to experience long periods of behavioural immobility with co-incidental changes in brain electrical activity (Nitz and Tononi, 2002).

Other insects are more problematic, trying to measure activity in sleeping bees is understandably difficult but at night they have been observed hanging onto a leaf with their jaws, legs folded up into their body, till morning when they fly away only to return to the same place the next evening.

Sleep is 250 million years old?

The excitement of discovering Rapid Eye Movement during sleep led many a tired scientist to give up their own bed to stare at the closed eyelids of slumbering animals. Some without success, as amphibians and fish have never been found to experience REM sleep.
Not surprising, as fully functional REM sleep is specific to warm blooded animals which means reptiles don't experience REM except for crocodiles who curiously do. However the electrical activity in crocodiles' brain is different from mammalian REM so it is assumed that crocodiles exhibit a prototype of REM sleep which may one day provide clues to the origin of REM.

Birds experience brief episodes of REM for about 5% of their total sleep cycle which lasts between ten to fifteen minutes. Scientists are uncertain as to why these periods are so short but birds, like aquatic mammals, also demonstrate 'unihemispheric' sleep - the ability to sleep with one half of the brain while the other half remains alert. Which may well indicate that both they and birds have to be alert virtually 24/7 to avoid predation.

However, REM sleep is such a necessary evil that, despite having reduced each segment to the barest minimum, modern birds still have had to make two evolutionary adaption's to cope.
The first involved turning the big toe (the hallux) backward, leaving the other three pointing forward, so that the four toes form a circle around a branch. During sleep birds normally perch on one foot and, even though they have better control of their body muscles than us, in the muscle relaxed state of REM sleep they could literally fall of their perch. So their secondary adaption was a special tendon stretching from toe to the thigh which retracts as the knee bends, curling toes tight around the bough to prevent them falling off during REM.

Discussing bird-sleep is relevant because birds evolved from dinosaurs and as the latest evidence suggests that dinosaurs were warm blooded, this could indicate that the full REM sleep function preceded the mammalian stage and evolved at least as far back as the dinosaurs. Further it has been suggested that the reason for its development in Crocodylidae is that they spend most of their lives in Equatorial Rivers,which maintain a constant tepid temperature, hence the reason for their possible development of an embryonic REM sleep state. It may also pinpoint REM sleep's evolution to the time when they split from dinosaurs approximately 250 million years ago.

The origins of REM

By 110 million years ago, mammals had diverged into two distinct groups, the marsupial mammals and the placental mammals as both groups display symptoms of advanced slow-wave sleep together with REM sleep, it indicates that REM sleep evolved at least one hundred and fifty years ago. So scientists hunting the origins of REM sleep began by looking at the oldest surviving mammals.

There are two such species, the duck billed platypus found in Australia and New Guinea and the echidnas which are unique to New Guinea. Both are primitive egg laying, toothless mammals

When the British Museum received the first stuffed platypus, in 1798, they thought it was a product of a fevered imagination.

Claiming that someone had sewed a ducks bill and a beaver's tail onto the body of an otter. Scottish zoologist Robert Knox was so incensed he took a pair of scissors to its skin looking for stitches.

But what most disturbed them were the claims from Australians that platypuses and echidnas laid eggs rather than giving birth to live young. The mystery was only solved eighty six years later in 1884, by another Scot, William Caldwell a postgraduate student, who with the help of Aborigines rounded up a number of platypuses on the Burnet River in northern Queensland and discovered a female, who had just laid one egg and had a second egg dilated in her uterus.

These primitive traits led scientist to believe that Monotremes' ancestors may have existed alongside the dinosaurs and so it was assumed they could give an indication as to the origins of REM sleep.

Early research found that there was no indication of the low voltage- high frequency brainwaves indicative of REM sleep in humans, either in Echidnae or Platypus . So scientists believed that REM sleep was not part of the monotremes' sleep cycle and therefore it must have evolved later than the Monotremes original ancestor i.e. less than one hundred million years ago.

But this hypothesis began to be questioned when instruments became more sensitive and it was first discovered that Echidnae (who sleep above ground permanently), do experience REM sleep but have learned to conceal signs of REM (more later), as a survival mechanism.

Then in 1998 J. M. Siegel et al., Department of Physiology and Pharmacology, University of Queensland, published an important paper, 'Monotremes and the evolution of rapid eye movement,' which revealed that the platypus not only displays REM brain activity whilst sleeping but experiences a massive 90% of its sleep in REM, which, more than any other animal.

Flip Flop v Fusion

And there was another significant differences. Instead of displaying the low voltage cortical arousal seen in REM sleep in modern mammals; Platypus experienced moderate as well as high-voltage cortical EEG's at the same time.

As neither their REM sleep duration nor their brain-wave emissions are the same as modern mammals, this led to the suggestion that in Monotremes the Delta waves of slow-wave sleep (which are high voltage,) fuse together with the relaxed muscle state of REM sleep with their lower voltage..

This would account for the difference in cortical arousal and explain the length of time (14hrs), they spend in sleep. Presumably the platypus is to a certain extent both brain dormant and muscle relaxed at the same time, which places it in the most vulnerable state of all and could explain why it rests in burrows.

This vulnerability could also explain why mammalian sleep evolved into separate segments; i.e. REM and slow-wave sleep diverged from the original 'fused' sleep state, so that the animal had an increased chance of waking if under threat.

Flip Flop v Fusion

As always in evolution there is more than one way of skinning a cat and in 2011, John Lesku et al., published a study funded by the Max Planck Institute for Ornithology entitled 'Ostriches Sleep like Platypuses,' which gave the first description of brain activity during sleep in ostriches.

The relevance may not prove to be as weird as it first sounds because the Ostrich is another 'archaic' animal and the research showed that their sleep activity is similar to that of the Monotremes but with one crucial difference. Ostrich REM sleep duration is greater than any other bird, and although they do exhibit rapid eye movement and reduced muscle tone theirs is not a fused state, as in the monotremes, instead they segregate the two states by flipping rapidly between slow-wave sleep and REM sleep.

The refinement of 'flip flopping' can be seen in modern birds today.

In 2008, Philip Low at the Salk Institute for Biological Sciences in La Jolla, California, US, monitored five zebra finches during the night, tracking their eye and body movements and brain activity.

They found that the birds displayed some of the characteristics of mammalian sleep - including REM periods and K-complexes - even though they lack a neocortex, common to higher mammals.

However their slow-wave sleep and REM sleep cycle occurred approximately every 10-15 minutes as opposed to our much own longer cycle, which presumably makes them less vulnerable to predators.

REM sleep in mammals

Although the research showed little evidence of sleep spindles, the presence of K-complexes suggests that birds have evolved, in common with mammals, the same mechanism to prevent audio disruption.
It also demonstrates a) how crucial it is to keep the animal quiescent during sleep and b) indicate that K-complexes may have evolved at an earlier stage than sleep spindles.

However as zebra finches phases of REM and Slow wave sleep are approximately there must be a channel of communication between them , so it is possible that either scientists haven't managed to detect any sleep spindles as yet, or birds have evolved a separate mechanism for carrying information between REM and slow wave sleep.
Whatever the device, modern birds have demonstrated that by separating and extending the periods they spend in each sleep state it is more efficient than 'flip flopping' between them, as they spend less than half the time in total sleep than ostriches.
Currently we can demonstrate that REM and slow wave sleep existed as a fused state in monotremes, up to 100 million years ago. Then approximately 20 million years ago ostriches had taken the step of separating the states and 'flip flopped' between them'. Sometime later mammals, and to a certain extent birds, devised a different method of separating
REM and slow wave sleep into smaller, compartmentalised, segments connected by sleep spindles. Couple this with the evidence that there has been little in the way of species radiation in platypus since they evolved, makes it possible that their single 'fused' sleep state evolved as early as the Dinosaurs which may give an indication as to how long Dinosaurs spent in sleep - nice to imagine a snoring T.rex.

REM sleep in Mammals
A study published in the European Journal of Wildlife Research 2008, found that Red deer resting bouts were shorter during the night than during the day from June to October. In other words Red deer took advantage of sleeping during the longer light conditions. Wildlife film makers assumed big cats did so too as most of their documentaries showed lions lazing asleep in the sun only rousing to make a desultory kill. But the invention of night vision cameras told a different story, completely disproving conventional wisdom; they revealed that the big cats hunt mainly at night. The reason is that as ruminants spend most of their daylight hours browsing they have to sleep at some time during the night. Which means predators may use the dark, not only for cover, but because they are more likely to surprise at least one animal in the paralysis of REM. Which perhaps explains why Red deer adapted to 'sleeping with the enemy?'

REM napping

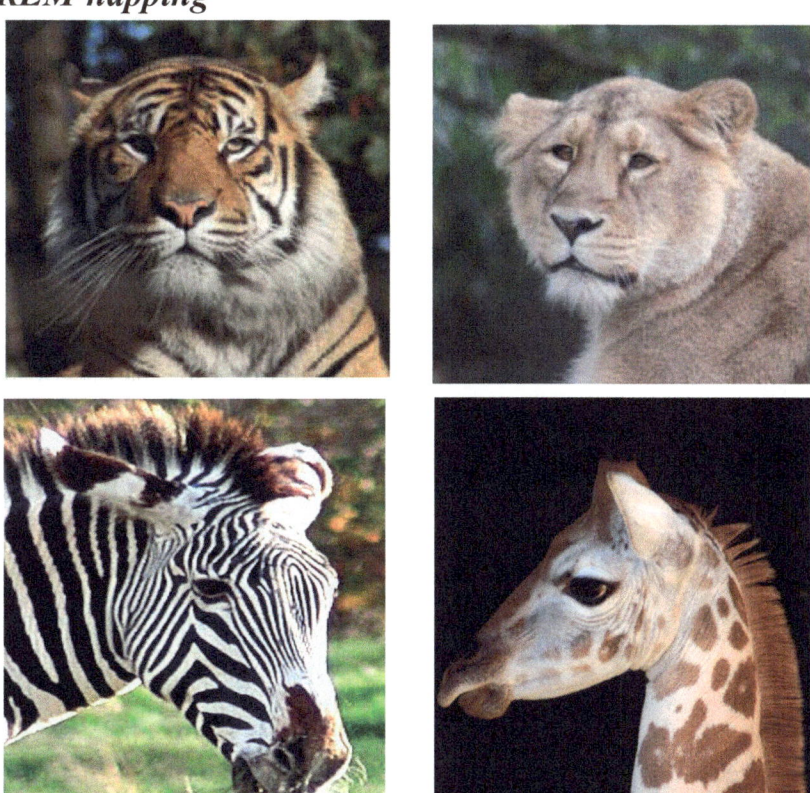

This delicate balance in the predator prey-war is evidenced by the evolution of white markings under and sometimes around the eyes to enhance 'night vision' and is a certain indication that the big cats and some herbivores are active at night. In the sample illustrations above, the white markings are clearly defined.

Not surprisingly Nature also evolved REM 'napping', a mechanism which limits time spent in REM to increase the chances of escape. There is no better demonstration of this than the correlation between the reduction of time spent in REM and the speed of a species specific predator, such as the Thompson Gazelle, who spend only four minutes at a time in REM and are predated on by the fastest land mammal the cheetah.
Sheep, on the other hand, can afford to sleep four times longer, because they live in herds which contain many eyes and sheep have evolved a 'sphinx like' sleeping posture i.e. front legs straight out below drooping head and neck. Although it looks odd it is the perfect position to gain a standing start if surprised by a predator (try creeping up on one and see how fast they get to their feet).

Carnivores are not generally under threat (except from us and the odd buffalo), whilst prey species, including birds, need to be constantly on their guard and, as already stated, reduce their need for sleep, particularly REM sleep when their skeletal muscles are paralysed. The more alert you are the readier to flee predation and the more chance you have of survival.

REM 'napping' is therefore based on perfectly sound biological and evolutionary reasons as it limits the periods spent in a 'frozen ' state, making it easier for prey species to respond to danger.

If for example we remained comatose for one continuous two and a half hour period of REM sleep every night., I doubt we would be here as a species.

Which is perhaps why the majority of archaeological evidence relating to Homo sapiens is found mainly in caves.

Carnivores like the big cats spend up to fourteen hours every day sleeping. Understandably there isn't much in the way of Lion REM research but presumably they are similar to domestic cats in that their 40% REM sleep total is higher than most ruminants (and humans), which averages 24%.

As many domestic cats sleep of a night with their owners, it may be worth comparing how much time they spend sleeping in the day (approximately six hours) to see if they have altered their sleeping habits to coincide with ours. If they sleep for longer than six hours between you getting up and going to bed then it's likely they are on the prowl at night. Most pedigree cats have had their markings altered by inbreeding but if you Google image a Scottish wild cat you will see the tell tale lighter markings under the eyes of their larger relatives.

Although these statistics may seem a trifle irrelevant the differences in sleep patterns between predators and prey, particularly their duration of REM sleep, is constant across the mammalian kingdom. Therefore REM's function must be absolutely critical to life otherwise Nature wouldn't have had to make such big compromises, particularly in prey-animal life styles, to accommodate it. Presumably this is why most mammals enjoy Polyphasic sleep (multiple bouts), whilst we and the great apes are monophasic i.e. we sleep for one single session averaging eight hours per night. On the face of it a dangerous occupation only explained by apes nesting in trees and, as stated, Homo sapiens preference for caves.

However, no matter if it be polyphasic or monophasic, we all undergo sleep, and we still need to discover why nature has taken such huge steps to accommodate REM sleep. But before we do, it may be worth examining the evidence for another adaption of the sleep process. The existence of REM sleep in marine mammals, which is sketchy to say the least.

Hemispherical sleep

The latest research indicates that their sleep cycle approximates with ours i.e. eight hours in every twenty four, but the situation is complicated because sea mammals have two brain hemispheres which allow one hemisphere to stay conscious whilst the other side is sleeping.

This curious phenomena known as hemispherical sleep is explained by a very necessary adaption as whales and dolphins need to surface regularly to breathe, which would be difficult underwater if their muscles were frozen in REM.

Both whales and dolphins are descendants of the 'Pakicetidae', meaning 'Pakistani whales'- a peculiar description for a small carnivorous land mammal which evolved only 55 million years ago.

However, as REM sleep may have evolved in land mammals up to 100 million years before whales and dolphins evolved, it is reasonable to assume that cetaceans do experience REM sleep.

This means that unlike birds, who also use hemispherical sleep and still experience REM paralysis, their adaption somehow managed to suppress the effects of REM paralysis.

Interestingly, in the year 2000, researchers, at the University of California at Santa Cruz, reported that a group of Pacific white-sided dolphins had been observed slowly swimming in a circle with one eye open (presumably controlled by the alert hemisphere), facing each other. Despite its 'Fantasia' imagery, it is probably the size of the group which prevents predator attack because as soon as sleep ceased the pod broke up to return to its normal activity. Perhaps the expression 'sleeping with one eye open' has more than a ring of truth to it.

* There have been no reports of land mammals (including us), ever exhibiting hemispherical sleep but as it is common to both birds and dolphins presumably it evolved pre 50 million years ago and early forms may have arisen with the dinosaurs.

,
Function of REM sleep.

In a study published in the 2008 journal of Human Brain Mapping, human participants were monitored with MRI imaging designed to visualize brain activity whilst in REM sleep. Researchers found activity in areas of the brain that control sight, hearing, smell, touch, balance and body movement including male erections.

And this is a clue to one of the tasks of REM sleep which is to 'test run' your body's vital functions. In this case it is 'wedding tackle', as some comedians call the crucial mechanism for continuing our genetic heritage.

Clinicians use these findings to check the basis for male erectile dysfunction (ED).

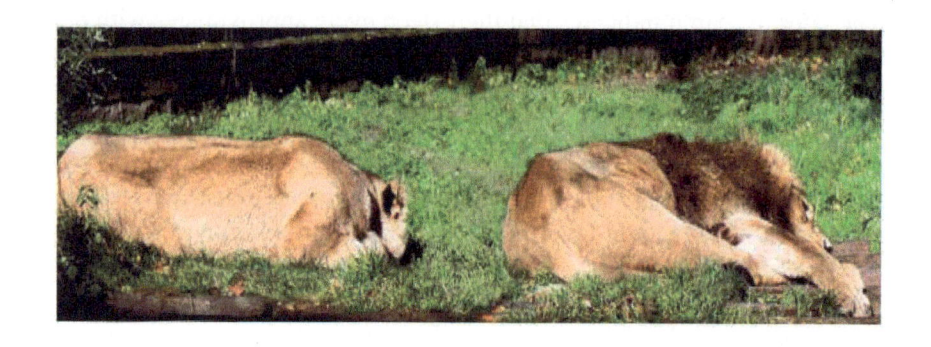

"In the jungle, the mighty jungle, the lion sleeps...to-day"

With apologies to the descendants of Solomon Linda

Function of REM sleep

If ED occurs whilst awake, but there is no dysfunction during REM sleep it is likely that ED is due to a psychological rather than a physiological cause. I was not clear as to how this was tested until I discovered that an elastic band is attached, last thing at night, which they hope to find broken in the morning. But the question still has to be asked, is this sufficient grounds for knocking us unconscious and put us at risk of predation? If so the reason must be vital... and it is.

In 1967 Michel Jouvet found a brain area in cats near a structure called the 'locus coeruleus' which is necessary for muscle relaxation during REM sleep. When this area was (regrettably) surgically destroyed the animals went to sleep normally but during REM sleep they ran around the cage with closed eyes hissing and scratching as if fighting with another animal.
Jouvet said, "The sleeping animal's behaviour may even be so fierce as to make the experimenter recoil." Which led him to this significant insight:

"Might deep muscle relaxation be necessary to prevent the animals from acting out their dreams and damaging themselves?"

At last we had a possible explanation as to why mammals (including us), are immobilised during REM sleep and here is where the original ideas relating sleep to dreaming still muddies the picture. We are not acting out a part in a surreal movie we are acting out something far deadlier and serious. Mammals don't lie down during REM sleep because they prefer too, the simple truth is they have no other option as their skeletal muscles are so relaxed they won't support them standing up! Even horses who have evolved a complex mechanism of tendons and ligaments that lock the knee cap, called a 'stay apparatus,' remain upright whilst in Slow wave sleep but if kept standing for long enough collapse when they enter REM sleep.
Giraffes, huge creatures that they are, REM sleep in one to six minute blocks over a 4.6 hour period but as it must be a real pain having to stagger to their feet they also mix sleep with an alert state at night so they can chew cud while lying down.
Cats sleep in an upright position during Non-REM sleep and lie down when they are in REM. Caring owners think their pets are dreaming when their body muscles occasional jerk, or 'twitch'. Unfortunately the signs are far from it; instead their treasured pets are demonstrating REM sleep leakage (muscle control inhibition leakage), the spasmodic return of muscle control as they desperately practise their fighting skills. Common to all mammals, REM-leakage can take various forms; chimpanzees howl, horse's neigh and dogs whimper.
*previous page two lions in REM

"As I recall I was in a dark and dusty house with cobwebs everywhere and as I got tangled in a hanging web, a large spider fell out of the web on to my neck and I woke up thrashing about to dislodge it."

Phil Cantlay

REM-leakage

In humans REM leakage can escalate to R.B.D (REM behaviour disorder), where the dreamer becomes violent, kicking, screaming, punching and sometimes jumping out of bed. Unfortunately often injuring themselves and their partner in the process. When woken, individuals recall the 'dream', together with its activities but most are unaware that they were physically moving, which is in direct contrast to sleepwalking as the individuals concerned have no recollection of what they were doing. This is confirmed by my oldest friend Phil Cantlay (born on the same day in the same ward as me,) who is the only person I know with R.B.D.
He told me that he recently dreamed he was being attacked by a spider and awoke as he was vigorously swiping it away.

Combining the 'aggressive' evidence from R.B.D together with Jouvet's 'cat' experiments make it most likely that one of the functions of REM sleep is dedicated to physically acting out some form of vigorous 'life saving' behaviour, such as cats defending themselves and platypus practicing swimming movements (next page). But most important of all, by freezing the body's skeletal muscles REM ensures that the behaviour happens without risk of personal or 'collateral' damage.
In the light of this, the expression ."Why don't you go and have a nice lie down," takes on a totally different meaning, as a) you have no option but to lie down and b) lying down in REM is anything but a nice experience. However, at last we have a good reason to explain why we are all muscle-bound during REM sleep and can refute the common held view that REM sleep is the time of night when we all go to the movies to watch surreal films, because REM sleep is when we act out crucial survival behaviours. But this only provokes more questions, e.g. what behaviours are we acting out and if so are they the same ones repeated every night, or do they change?

The interaction between Slow wave sleep and REM.
In 2001, Matthew A. Wilson, associate professor of brain and cognitive sciences in MIT's Picower Center for Learning and Memory, conducted a series of experiments which showed for the first time the relationship between slow-wave sleep and REM sleep. With biology graduate student Kenway Louie they trained rats to run along a circular track for a food reward. As each animal ran they recorded the pattern of neurons firing in its hippocampus. When they monitored the animals during REM sleep episodes they discovered that approximately 50% of the rats repeated the unique signature of brain activity they created when they ran round the track.

Interaction of S.W.S & REM

What turned out to be highly significant was that this not only confirmed the 'acting out' function as suggested by Jouvet, but it also revealed that REM sleep brain activity took approximately the same time to complete as the live situation.

Presumably this is a more efficient way for a rat to commit its behaviour to memory as its brain will be too busy during the journey with the distractions of finding the best route. More efficient to wait until it has completed the task then re-run the successful route, whilst the brain is quiescent, and pass on the results for REM to save as mind-map for future reference into its personal cognitive Sat Nav.

Matthew Wilson's next study, conducted with co-author brain and cognitive sciences graduate student Albert K. Lee, focussed on the effects of the same experiment on slow-wave sleep.

Two astonishing aspects of their findings stood out; a) Similar results were achieved but they were replayed at very high speed during slow-wave sleep, i.e. a four-second lap replayed in only 100/200 milliseconds in other words at approximately 40x.

b) Although hippocampal reactivation was detected in the cortex during all sleep sessions (which further supports the theory that sleep is involved in regulating our memory processes),slow-wave sleep replay was most robust during the sleep period immediately following alert behaviour and was not detectable 24 hours later. This would suggest that the new day's memories are the first to be sorted by slow wave sleep before they are forwarded to the first and second phases of REM (see chart p35) to be embedded as long term memories into our frontal cortex. Which ties in neatly with the findings of the Berkley study (page 26) of the students who slept for ninety minutes (which includes the first phase of REM),before waking with literally more room in the memory bin (the hippocampus) to remember new information.

The question. "If both slow-wave sleep and REM sleep exist as separate segments, neither fused together nor sharing a flip flop scenario then how do they communicate with each other?" Is answered by the University of California, Berkeleys study which suggested that sleep spindles move fact-based memories from the 'limited ' storage space of the brain's hippocampus to the prefrontal cortex.

Further if we use Turing's logic and look at the Berkeleys results in reverse by putting the slow wave sleep findings first i.e. "Slow wave sleep replay was most robust in the first period of slow wave sleep." It indicates that slow wave sleep is the first to be activated by sleep spindles carrying information from the hippocampus.

Sleep Cycle Mechanism

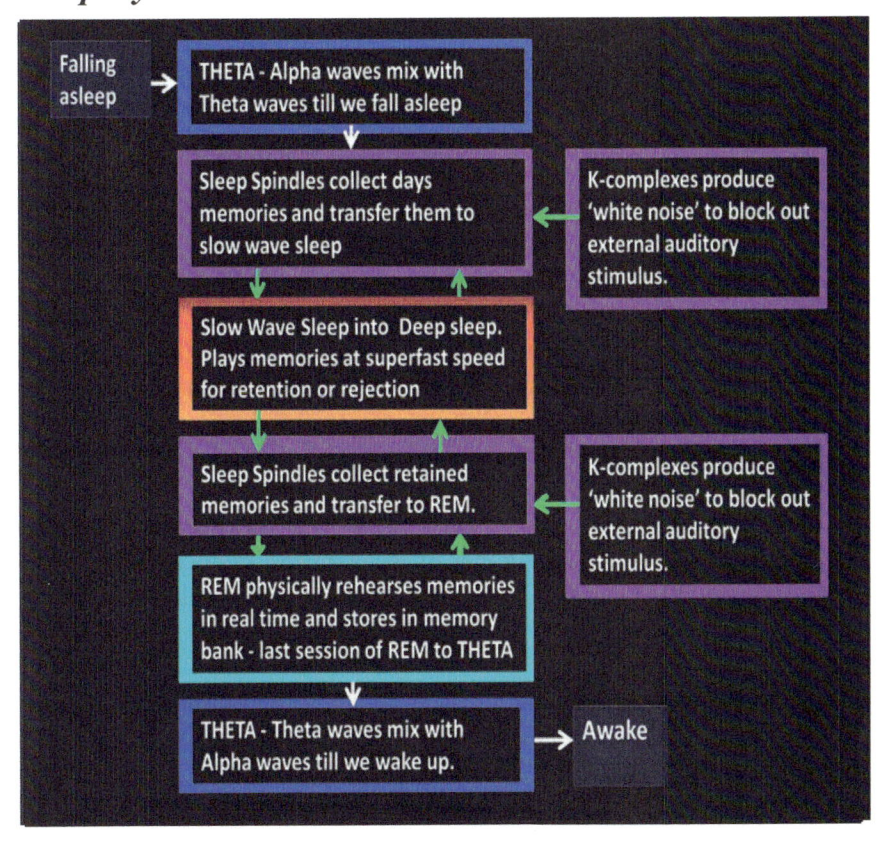

```
Falling asleep → THETA - Alpha waves mix with Theta waves till we fall asleep
    ↓
Sleep Spindles collect days memories and transfer them to slow wave sleep  ←  K-complexes produce 'white noise' to block out external auditory stimulus.
    ↓ ↑
Slow Wave Sleep into Deep sleep. Plays memories at superfast speed for retention or rejection
    ↑
Sleep Spindles collect retained memories and transfer to REM.  ←  K-complexes produce 'white noise' to block out external auditory stimulus.
    ↑
REM physically rehearses memories in real time and stores in memory bank - last session of REM to THETA
    ↓
THETA - Theta waves mix with Alpha waves till we wake up.  →  Awake
```

Therefore it would be logical to assume that Slow wave sleep and hence Deep sleep is instrumental in sorting out new memories, for rejection or retention, before passing the memories worth saving over to REM, via sleep spindles.

Doing so at high speed, not only saves 'vulnerable time' in Deep sleep but leaves REM less work to do so it can afford to replay and reorganise memories, in real time, (which would also explain, from Rem leakage evidence why Phil's behaviour , swatting away a spider, occurred in real time.) In other words this is how the day's memories are organised; junk memories are dumped whilst useful memories are passed onto the REM stage to be consolidated into permanent memories by 're-enactment'.

The objective, neatly encapsulated by Alan Dunn's image of a memory card on a pillow, is to empty the hypothalamus of memories so it can store new ones the next day.

Each night we fight for our lives

With one further refinement, before they are uploaded, slow wave sleep sorts out the junk before it sends the critical memories to be saved by REM sleep. No one knows, as yet, how the 'selection process operates' but we can deduct how they are stored (later). Nor do we understand the undoubted other cognitive or physical 'repair' processes that are also being directed by the brain at the same time.

Nevertheless now that we have a rudimentary idea as to the mechanism we can explain why sleep spindles take up the majority of the total sleep cycle, because they have to transmit the information more than once; i.e. first to slow wave sleep before again ferrying saved memories over to REM.
Scientists have speculated that up to 95 percent of our day's experiences are disposed of during slow-wave sleep.
This makes sense if you think about all the useless information your brain is constantly taking in. The number of faces, buses, taxis, cars, etc., you see on an everyday journey - if you retained them all it would soon jam up your cognitive functioning.

Wilson's evidence also explains why we can't recall all those short term memories, as after 24hours there is no way to 'undelete' the recycle bin. It's emptied every night... when they're gone they're gone.
And although the selection process is not understood it is crucial for our survival. Think how difficult it would be if the wrong memories were dumped everynight.Trying to find your way to work as if it were your first day, everyday, over and over again... no need for the film Groundhog Day"!

Getting rid of unwanted memories is easy to understand its the physically acting out the retained ones that is, for me, hard to understand.
However, bearing in mind Jouvet's 'cat fight' observations and the violence involved in human REM behaviour disorder, it seems that REM sleep is indeed a primal mechanism which probably evolved in excess of 250 million years ago to embed successful defence strategies into waking behaviour.

What better time to use the adage 'practice makes perfect' than in your sleep, if you try it in a real live situation you may not survive to use it again. This tallies with the length of time carnivores Big Cats spend in REM as they spend far more awake time not only play fighting but developing team skills when they stalk prey, which all has to be rehearsed in REM.

Perhaps it would be worthwhile to pause and take stock for a moment:
* It must be stressed that Brainwaves also perform a multitude of other physiological functions during sleep,which means that although the research neatly divides sleep-stages into a brain wave segment,it only refers to their pre-dominance i.e there is never 100%. produced at any one time.

* The chart on page 36 is a simplistic construction which only shows the stages and not the length of time spent in each segment. An idea of duration can be gained by referring to the illustrations on pages 23-24-25.

* My friend Phil told me that recently he fell asleep for five minutes on the couch and woke up flailing his arms, which means he was obviously in REM (displaying leakage). This could explain why some men fall asleep in the day, as getting up in the night interrupts the sleep process and a REM segment still needs to consolidate the information transferred to it by sleep spindles.

*If your thinking og getting a dog rather than a burglar alarm, consider this: All mammals undergo the same stages of sleep as ourselves, which means that canines can sleep through a break-in!

* Scary as it may seem, all of us, from childhood to old age, including dignitaries and celebrities, spend a large part of the night fighting for our lives! Perhaps it's a good job that nature has made sleep so seductively pleasant and we have little memory of the process.

* If you follow the' 24 stages of sleep' chart on page 36, it is significant that there are only two segments of Deep sleep. And as we have already seen, from Matthew A. Wilson's results, it is likely that they are involved in sorting out the days new memories which are rehearsed during the next two periods of REM. Which means that older, pre-existing survival strategies are rehearsed during the last three periodsof REM. If it were possible to correlate details of remembered REM leakage activities, together with the time they occurred, it may well shed further light on the matter.

* Recently I met a man, whose vision has been deteriorating throughout his life and now he has practically none. He told me that no matter how many sleeping tablets he took, he could only sleep for four hours every night. Further his sleep periods had shortened in conjunction with his sight deterioration. We inevitably discussed this book and he suddenly said, "I know why I can only sleep for four hours, it's because my brain doesn't have to process any visual information!" This not only makes perfect sense but has also been confirmed by another visually impaired person.

REM sleep segments total two hours compared to None-REM sleep which totals between four and six hours. This confirms that sleep spindles and slow-wave sleep have a lot more work to do, sorting out the relevant memories from the unwanted ones, so it comes as no surprise that 95% are junk As yet, nobody knows what criteria are used to ditch or save memories, but it is significant that the reduction in duration of REM and slow wave sleep segments in modern mammals (compared to platypus) is also accompanied by sleep spindles. Which, as they don't exist in either the monotremes, 'fused' sleep state or the Ostriches, 'flip flop' state, indicates they are the latest step in sleep evolution. Conversely, rapid eyeball movements during sleep is common to all modern mammals and birds and also exists in monotremes, so it would suggest that REM is older than 100 million years. Which further supports the theory that REM and slow wave sleep are the 'critical' segments and sleep spindles are simply a faster way of communicating between them.

This brings us to the question, "If REM sleep is critical then does that mean that rapid eyeball movement and 'dreaming' are critical too?"

Is dreaming simply fragmented recollections of REM, or is it connected with the eyes watching a dream?

Part of the question is answered by another. As rapid eyeball movement is fast and jerky and REM sleep plays out in real time. Would it not be more appropriate to the helter-skelter speed of Deep sleep?

To attempt to answer these questions we need to first look at the function of eye movement in humans which is best demonstrated by those of us who cannot see.

Eye movement during communication

Watch any person blind from birth talking (You Tube) and you will note that their eyes move constantly, almost involuntarily as they speak.

It can be disconcerting until you observe a sighted person speaking and notice that their eyes also move, albeit in a more controlled manner.

When two people are conversing over coffee, for example, the listener looks at the speaker for about seventy five percent of the time. Interestingly the behaviour has been constantly reinforced from childhood particularly by teachers insisting ... "Look at me when I'm talking to you."

This is because the speaker needs to know that they are being listened too and they check by looking at the listener for twenty five percent of the time to ensure they still have their full attention. This leads to a visual dance as the speaker's eyes alternate between looking at the listener and moving away from the listener.

55.

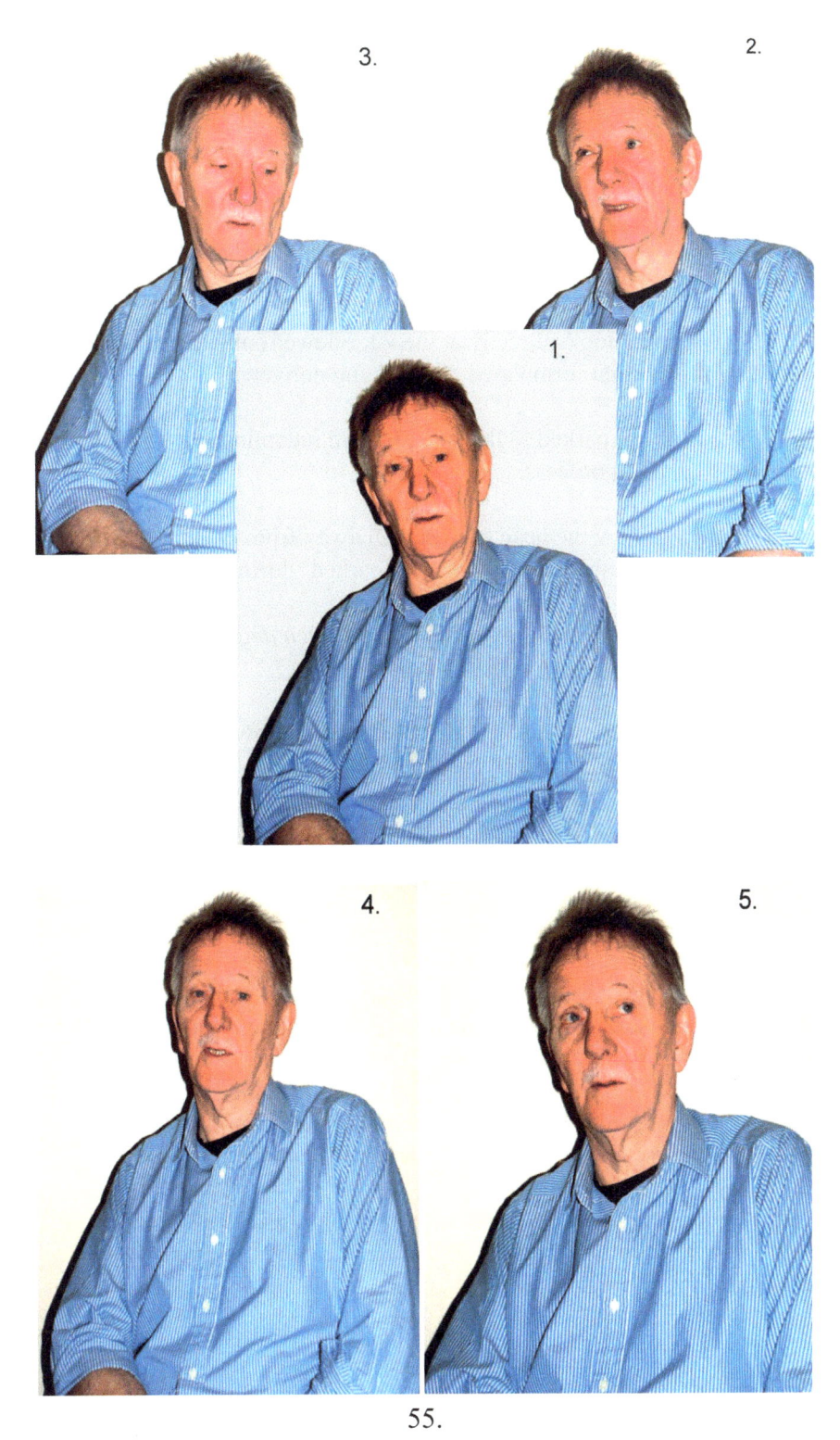

Eye movement during communication

Keep watching for long enough and a clear pattern emerges between eye movement and speech. The speaker's eyes slide away from the listener a split second before they offer new information. This shift in eye gaze prior to verbalisation is so important that it is often reinforced by the head turning away as well.

The illustrations, left, show the synchrony of eye and head movement during a conversation.

No 1. The speaker looks directly at the interviewer only after the new information has been formulated and is being delivered.

No 2. The eyes are parked to the side to avoid incoming information during the thinking process.

No 3. Indicates how the head can tilt well away from the centre with varying degrees of shift, as the eyes are 'parked' during thinking.

* Research might establish a correlation between degree of head movement and complexity of the thought process.

No 4. Although the subject appears to be looking towards the interviewer, the eyes are out of focus.

No 5. The eyes are parked again but in the opposite direction to No 2.

So, why do we move our eyes whilst thinking and talking? The answer is quite simple; the brain can't cope with storing information at the same time as extracting it. In other words it is not possible to take in visual information at the same time as co-ordinating our thought processes. Blinking is also unique to Homo sapiens, our average 'blink rate' is far more than required to simply 'wipe' the eyeballs and is a neat way of allowing us to keep visually focused on a subject whilst we retrieve information in short bites. Evolved, presumably, to minimise the problem of being unable to retrieve and assimilate information simultaneously.

Test it by focussing on the object your eyes are directed towards whilst your thinking. It totally disrupts your train of thought because you brain stops the current thought process to deal with the incoming visual stimulus.

Which means that if a person keeps looking directly at you, whilst their talking itmeans that their speech has been rehearsed i.e. it is NOT spontaneous. Bit difficult to believe but ask anyone a familiar question and watch their response compared to an unfamiliar one. Or observe a politician on T.V. and see how their eyes fix on the interviewer when they're on solid ground i.e. the well rehearsed party line. However, if they are asked an unsettling question their eyes will move sideways before they answer. Thus accounting for the possibly unfair association in Western society, that eye movement equals untrustworthiness ..."they look shifty to me." When all it indicates is the person is thinking.

Perhaps it is also why people who don't tell the truth are advised to have good memories, in other words to rehearse their stories so they can, "Look you straight in the eye." But being 'looked in the eye' whilst a person is talking is only evidence of a rehearsed thought, be it true or untrue.

Which leads to a further argument against the use of phones, both in-car and mobile, whilst driving. "If a drivers eyes are unfocused whilst their thinking about their reply during a phone conversation, then how can they process the visual information they are being presented with at high speed?" In fact, should a conversation take place between a passenger and driver at all?
Blocking out visual stimulus, whilst the brain assesses a particular piece of information is common to all mammals. Bulls roll their eyes back whilst sniffing a potential mate for pheromones; wolves do the same as their heads go up to howl; lesser apes eyes flicker briefly as they chitter to each other even Koko the talking gorilla (famous for her sign language skills), only moves her eyes fractionally, when 'communicating' with her instructors. Although these eye movements indicate that the animal is 'thinking' i.e. it is searching for an appropriate response to a situation from its stored memories (wolves replaying a rehearsed song, lesser apes vocalising learned communication responses), they are only doing so from a script based on past experience, they are not constructing 'new thoughts'. Which, as we shall discuss later, is related to intelligence not Imagination.

As all races of man, both sighted and non-sighted, use eye movement during conversation it a) indicates that eye movement during speech is genetically governed and b) that thinking behaviour must have evolved at an early stage in our own evolution. But what is really important in our pursuit of the evolution of Imagination is that 'eye movement during speech' is a further development of the same cognitive processes that evolved in mammals i.e. it is only a development, not a completely new mutation!

Dr Doollitle sang;

> "*I conferred with our furry friends, man to animal,*
> *Think of the amazing repartee*
> *If I could walk with the animals, talk with the animals,*
> *Grunt and squeak and squawk with the animals,*"
>
> Perhaps he should have added...
> "*Ah, but could they talk to me?*"

For animal communication has a finite limit and is restricted to relaying simple messages; danger, fear, mating-calls;ect, whereas human verbal communication not only relies on 'set responses' but is infinitely variable and requires much more cognitive reflection before delivery, which accounts for our, comparatively, extreme use of eye movement.

Which, as discussed, is further evidence that our thought processes are a unique evolutionary adaption and the construction of abstract thought appears to be exclusive to us.

Notes on p 56-58.

* *Recently researchers discovered that each time a persons eyes look 30 degrees upwards, the brain produces a short, quick burst of Alpha brain waves. This is important as we also know that Alpha waves are generated during Theta, REM and Slow wave sleep, as well as our conscious state. So it very much looks as if Alpha waves are common to the function of our cognitive processes and as we shall discover may well point to their role in Imagination.*

** *It is also apparent that actors seem to have the ability to use eye movement in the appropriate way when delivering their 'learned' lines. Whether this is due to instinct or coaching has yet to be investigated..*

** *Computers obey the same laws as they cannot send and receive an email at the same time .*

*"Are not the sane and the insane equal at night
as the sane lie a dreaming?"*

Charles Dickens -1859

Is sleep the death of each day's life?

Having discussed the role of brainwaves during sleep it is now time to examine the role of brain waves during our 'waking' periods.
In 1859, Charles Dickens came close to explaining the nature of Imagination when he published this article called 'Night Walks', in his weekly journal, 'All Year Round'.

"And the fancy was this:
Are not the sane and the insane equal at night as the sane lie a dreaming? Are not all of us outside this hospital, who dream, more or less in the condition of those inside it, every night of our lives?

Are we not nightly persuaded, as they daily are, that we associate preposterously with kings and queens, emperors and empresses, and notabilities of all sorts? Do we not nightly jumble events and personages and times and places, as these do daily?

Are we not sometimes troubled by our own sleeping inconsistencies, and do we not vexedly try to account for them or excuse them, just as these do sometimes in respect of their waking delusions? Said an afflicted man to me, when I was last in a hospital like this, 'Sir, I can frequently fly.'

I was half ashamed to reflect that so could I-by night. Said a woman to me on the same occasion, 'Queen Victoria frequently comes to dine with me, and her Majesty and I dine off peaches and maccaroni in our night-gowns, and his Royal Highness the Prince Consort does us the honour to make a third on horseback in a Field-Marshal's uniform.'

Could I refrain from reddening with consciousness when I remembered the amazing royal parties I myself had given (at night), the unaccountable viands I had put on table, and my extraordinary manner of conducting myself on those distinguished occasions?

I wonder that the great master who knew everything (Shakespeare's Macbeth), when he called Sleep the death of each day's life, did not call Dreams the insanity of each day's sanity."

"Each day's sanity is the insanity of dreams"

The article by Dickens was based on many 'observational' walks round London and included the previous passage relating to his visit to Bethlehem Hospital, previously called Bedlam: His observations are acutely perceptive but if only he had said... "Each day's sanity is the insanity of dreams." He would have been much nearer the truth!
For how many of us have imagined being able to fly? Or daydreamed, "...that we associate preposterously with kings and queens, emperors and empresses, and notabilities of all sorts?"

In these difficult financial times many people have daydreamed (sometimes described as a reverie or 'lost in thought'), what they would do if they won the lottery by imagining living in a mansion and driving a Ferrari? Is this not the exact same phenomena experienced by the people Dickens termed insane? Both states involve recall of memories which are not necessarily based on our real life experiences but on things we have seen, which are then juxtapositioned with others to zoom in/out; including sound; emotion; dialogue, etc into our own unique film clip which we are personally directing.

The only difference is that daydreaming allows us to develop strategies for the future e.g. "I know exactly what I will do if I win the lottery." Whereas the inmates of Bedlam believed their fantasy was reality.

Test your own recall manipulation skills by remembering the last meeting you had with a friend for coffee. It should be easy to move from the coffee shop and imagine you are both holidaying together, first class ,on a yacht in the Caribbean, with the sun beating down and the wind flapping round your deckchair. You can also substitute your friend for a film star, sit next to them in the first class lounge bar, offer them a drink and discuss the possibility of you appearing in their next film. The sky's the limit because your brain is practising exactly what it is meant to do which is to manipulate memories and edit them into a new and logical sequence.

The result is exactly the same as dreaming. Except for one crucial difference, Daydreams are under our conscious control.
Given the complexity of our cognitive mechanisms daydreaming, has many functions, which have not been fully investigated, but one thing for sure is they allow us to experience the emotions of success even if there unachievable i.e. how many fans daydream about scoring the winning goal in the F.A. cup? As the saying goes "Were all entitled to dream." But 'entitled' is a misnomer for it suggests we are at liberty to decide to daydream or not, which is untrue.

Daydreaming is an active regulated process

Daydreaming, like sleep, is an active regulated process - it's something you can't prevent. Nor are they easy to measure, possiby because they are so innocuous it's difficult to consciously recognise them.

Try counting the number of times you slip into a reverie, even for a few seconds, during the day. Particularly when someone says something that triggers you into thinking about something else.

Scientists believe daydreaming is a natural mechanism triggered by the need to reduce strong emotions, i.e. 'revenge strategies'. Imagining the boss spilling soup down his/her front is a prime example.

Daydreaming is a warm up exercise.

This may well be, but if you strip daydreams of their content you are left with a mechanical process which has two distinct functions a) the selection of data (i.e. memories) and b) the manipulation of those memories into scenarios to enable you to select the one promising the best result. However as daydreaming arises spontaneously it could also be construed as a series of warm up exercises to keep your brains mechanical processes ticking over in 'standby' mode till you are ready to use them during 'deliberate' thinking In other words just as you can't prevent sleeping you can't stop daydreaming either.

Deliberate Thinking.

Thinking uses the total power of your imagination at full throttle.
All other senses are dimmed or switched off completely ("sorry I didn't hear you... I was thinking about something else."), as you busily run scenarios through your mind.

Some people relate it to computing power but this isn't simple number crunching. This is retrieval and comparison of data on an unimaginable scale in multi-sense dimensions, and that's before you start adding other factors in. Take the comparatively simple task of deciding where to eat out with a group of friends. Not only do you have to consider locations; menus; cost; ambiance ; friends food preferences; transport; etc, but each comparison can be accompanied by visual images, sound, smells, etc.

No wonder the brain exercises itself by daydreaming to keep the mechanical processes ready for use at any time. What also makes sense is that we don't have to constantly re-think a solution because the successful ones are embedded in our long term memory in the same way our practical experiences are at night.

Presumably Psychologists and Coaches also use the same mechanism to train sportsmen and women to 'think winning', in the hope that it becomes winning behaviour.

Daydreaming and Alpha waves

The system of 'practice makes perfect', devised long before the field of Sports Psychology, demonstrates that H. sapiens knew full well the benefits of rehearsing an activity, both physiologically and psychologically. What wasn't known was that REM sleep was the trainer! Scientists have also discovered that Daydreaming is accompanied by Alpha wave emissions centred in the occipital lobe (the visual processing centre at the rear of the brain), which is why some scientists believe we are able to visualise our day-dreams. Alpha waves are also emitted in REM sleep but they emanate from a totally different area in a frontal-central location in the brain. In both cases their purpose has not been explained but what is significant is that Alpha waves are not only common to REM sleep and daydreaming, but also to psychotic hallucinations (Dickens), and the hallucinations experienced when entering N1 (the Theta -drowsy sleep stage).

Consequently this commonality would lead to the obvious conclusion that the manipulation and replaying of memories is the responsibility of Alpha waves. The only difference is they carry out the same function in two totally different environments. During Daydreaming Alpha waves are under semi conscious control as the individual is still alert, and unlike REM sleep, their skeletal muscles and eyeballs, albeit out of focus, have full mobility. God knows what secrets that dark pool hold**s**.

Why do we remember Dreams?
Previously it was assumed that N1, the drowsy stage, was the key player in dreaming, as people only remembered their dreams when they woke in the morning. But back in the sixties researchers reported that people recalled dreaming whenever they were aroused from any one of the five REM segments.

Which means dreaming can have little to do with N1, as the drowsy stage only connects with the last segment of REM at the end of the sleep cycle. Nevertheless dreams are generally remembered when we wake up (except for those who say they never dream) and there are the occasional nightmares, which 'haunt' us for quite a while.

Taken together with 'bad' or 'broken' dreams (which people often attribute to eating certain types of food), the list of dream types is so extensive it has led many to make a fortune out of their interpretation. Yet nobody in the 'Dream industry' talks about the one factor common to all dreams and that is... their retention over time.

Perhaps the question can be first answered by asking."How long are your dreams remembered for?"

Why do we remember Dreams?

An hour; one day; a week; a month? The evidence is for as little as eight minutes! This is much longer than 'non-REM' dreams, which though rarely reported do occur and consist of fleeting fragmentary impressions that rarely contain visual imagery and are only remembered briefly when woken during slow wave sleep. Exactly the sort of recall you would expect from memories running at forty time's normal speed!

However, the evidence that dream memories fade so quickly indicates that they are not meant to be retained for conscious use. They have a much more serious purpose involving survival.

To date there is no research to indicate the total number of dreams we experience each night. Understandably it's hard to quantify, as we only remember a dream from whichever segment we wake from. But it does show we are 'dreaming' during each segment and if each REM segment acts out only one dream, in real time, then we only 'dream' five times a night.I find this difficult to believe, because the final period of REM lasts for one hour, which woulkd mean be one heck of a dream. Is it not more likely that we perform multiple re-enactments (dreams) and only remember the sequence we were re-enacting at the time we wake? Whatever, the evidence that we can remember 'only one dream' out of a minimum of five supports the theory that remembering dreams is not important, otherwise we would remember all of them.

What is the function of REM sleep and so called dreaming?

The evidence of REM leakage in all mammals indicates that dreaming, far from being a random event, has a definite purpose and one of its main functions is to practice survival behaviour.

This doesn't just involve fighting, fleeing or killing for food; it also includes survival of the species, as human REM leakage can involve performing the sex act during REM,which links in neatly with the evidence of nightly erections during REM.

It makes sense for REM to practice and 'make perfect' existing survival behaviour but as life is never static it would also make sense for it to attempt to provide solutions to any new problems encountered during the day. It is hardly likely that a killer spider is going to descend on my friend, Phill, in the U.K. But in his case he may have seen a spider in that day which, combined with memories of a scary film about spiders, prompted REM to act out a possible scenario to find a solution in case he meets a spider it in real life. However, as we all live in a social context it would also make sense if REM acted out 'social situations' as well.

Dreams in animals.

Recently I (a bit ashamedly), spoke to my hairdresser who I hadn't seen for a few months. He asked me what style I was growing my hair into? That night I dreamed I had a variety of hairstyles from Afro to punk to short back and sides which at my age, believe me, was quite disturbing. But it did lead me to wonder if it would be possible to analyse remembered dreams, in terms of 'issue resolution', using just three basic criteria. Are they about; surviving (fighting or fleeing); sexual strategies or social strategies? If so, it may well reveal a simple mechanism underlying their often bizarre form. It may also explain the phenomena of nightmares as a manifestation of an issue that REM can't resolve, e.g. were running away but still being pursued.
However even if we could analyse dreams in this way, the fact is we don't remember dreams on anything like a regular basis, so what use are they? Why undergo REM? Why dream? The answer could lie in the fact that REM sleep dates back at least one hundred million years (Echidnae), well before the evolution of Imagination, at a paltry one hundred thousand, or so. Which means they can have little to do with Imagination,so what use would remembered dreams be to animals, one hundred million years ago?

Further, if Imagination is the ability to recall and 'juggle' a series of different memories and run them to a logical conclusion to predict an outcome, then how would it help any animal who has to make a split second decision to save its life? Waiting to 'way up the situation' may prove fatal. Yes, animals do make behaviour selection by referring to memories during everyday living but not when it comes to survival, they act without waiting.
This perhaps is the key to understanding part of REM's function which is to convert rehearsal strategies into instinct Which would explain why we don't remember our dreams (by and large), we have no need, they go straight into our brains 'instinct survival' bank.
All the foregoing would be easily clarified if we could compare our human experience with dreaming in other animals. We know they experience REM sleep but there is no evidence to show if they display the emotional reaction one would associate with waking from a 'bad dream' (check your pet) and unfortunately we can't ask them. Also, most people still confuse REM leakage with animals remembering their dreams, as they think they are dreaming when they whimper or move. The only relevant research has been conducted on healthy laboratory animals (non-vivisection), mainly rats and cats, who when continuously deprived of sleep showed only impaired cognitive and body functions which eventually lead to their death.

Does an animal own its own body?

Back in 1959 Michel Jouvet also noted that, "Even during the longest deprivations, we have not seen hallucinatory-like behaviour such as described in cats with pontine lesions", which ties in with our discussion about hallucinations (and hence Imagination), being exclusively human and therefore not related to dreaming. It does raise another, some may side issue, which is relevant to our earlier discussion on airlines and sleep deprivation. When contestants in Channel 4's Big Brother programme in January 2004 where deprived of sleep for up to 120 hours. They experienced hallucinations, paranoia and disorientation which led some participants to describe the experience as 'torture'. A significant phrase, well illustrated by Menahem Begin ex Prime Minister of Israel who described his experience as a prisoner of the NKVD in Russia thus: "In the head of the interrogated prisoner, a haze begins to form. His spirit is wearied to death, his legs are unsteady, and he has one sole desire: to sleep... Anyone who has experienced this desire knows that not even hunger and thirst are comparable with it."

Sleep deprivation has been used for centuries as a means of interrogation, and it still continues in the 21st century, despite the European Convention of Human Rights: article 3. Which considers it "inhuman or degrading treatment or punishment."

However some unexpected results have emerged from Jouvet's and co's experiments. Animal Rights groups who fight continuously to secure humane treatment for animals have developed a new tactic to address a more fundamental issue. Does the animal own the right to its body?

In 2005 a Brazilian court was asked to grant an order of Habeas Corpus (determines if a person is imprisoned lawfully) in respect of a chimpanzee called Suica living in Salvador Zoo. The case was delayed because the judge wanted extra time to give serious consideration to the issue. Unfortunately Suica died before any ruling could be made.

Then in 2007 a case wishing to ascribe 'personhood' to a chimpanzee living in Austria named Mathew Hiasl Pan, was referred to the Europe Court of human rights.

In June 2009 the Spanish government was expected to recognise a law which gave great apes the right to life and also protect them from harmful research and from torture. As yet we still await an outcome for Mathew's case and to Spanish recognition of the law, but one wonders how any eventual ruling will affect the rights of animals in relation to Jouvet and co's experiments? If the animals do own their own body then their permission will have to be sought prior to captivity and experimentation... interesting.

Defragging the Brain.

Everything we experience; see; hear, taste, touch, smell i.e. 'encode' during our conscious existence, is recorded in memory. At the same time the brain is like a computer constantly opening, closing, saving, playing and manipulating memories, etc. We have already discussed the difficulty the brain has taking in information whilst it is retrieving it so it is hard to see how the brain can keep organising and filing memories in real time. It is more likely that the information quickly fragments spreading all over the brain's memory system like a child's bedroom after playtime with mum's carefully 'tidied' toys.
So it would make sense if the brain runs its own computer-like Defrag programme when its main functions are closed i.e. when it's asleep. This means the brain is then free to re-sort and categorises its memories to increase their later speed of retrieval and free up space for more efficient use.

Although we have discussed how slow wave and REM sleep carry out different memory related processes between them, no one knows how memories are categorised or stored by the brain.
However a series of further experiments conducted on rats by Matthew Wilson in 2006 concluded that their memories during sleep were co-ordinated into a series of time frames-which to me sound similar to Mpeg files.
This would make perfect sense as it is difficult to conceive how all the sensory information relating to a memory could be kept separately. Difficult trying to retrieve memories stored in separate 'sense' categories. Easier if memories could be stored like cognitive film clips, on You Tube ,which open with a still frame, till you press play.

But there the similarities end, for if you return to the meeting with your friend in a coffee shop, it isn't just an audio visual experience. You can also smell the coffee; fragrance of flowers on the table; remember the mood you were in; the weather at the time; you can shrink them to sit underneath a giant flower, change their clothes, facial expression, give them big ears, large noses, etc.
The combinations of memories are virtually limitless and totally validate Donald Rumsfeld's quote, while serving as United States Secretary of Defence, in February 2002:

"There are known known's; there are things we know that we know. There are known unknowns; that is to say there are things that, we now know we don't know. But there are also unknown unknowns. There are things we do not know we don't know."

Cognitive Youtube

With three billion people constantly manipulating their imagination many times a day, is it any wonder we have made such miraculous advancements as a species and is it any wonder that it is virtually impossible to totally predict the future (e.g. in 1999, would anyone have foreseen the impact of social media, or the fact that you have to buy a tank to traverse our cities so called 'speed bumps'), as there will always be 'things we do not know we don't know!"

The recall of memory detail in 3D, together with all the associated senses and emotions is almost limitless, light years ahead of any film or computer generated video. So the job of breaking down memories and storing them in separate categories i.e. sight, sound, smell, touch, etc. seems virtually impossible, particularly if you have to retrieve them in an instant.
Therefore Mathew Wilson's research, suggesting they are stored as a film clips, makes perfect sense.

The diagram on p34 illustrates that REM sleep is a busy period with its mix of Alpha and Beta waves. So we know that both waves are involved in the re-running of memories during REM.

However Alpha waves are not only present in REM but they are also present in slow wave sleep. Both states involved with playing memory clips. During our awake state Beta waves predominate but, according to the latest evidence, closed eyelids reduce the production of Beta waves and increase the production of Alpha waves. Further when we are day- dreaming Alpha waves predominate.

Therefore as Beta waves only predominate when we are taking in information. Would it not be reasonable to assume that Beta waves are responsible for storing the incoming information whilst Alpha waves are the mechanism which plays the 'movie clips'. Taking this view it looks as if during REM , Alpha waves are the DVD player mechanism which runs the memories received from slow wave sleep, as film clips, whilst Beta waves store them.

Similarly it would be impossible for daydreaming to function without being able to easily retrieve memories , so it makes further sense to assume that Beta waves as well as saving information also retrieve it from the same location it stored them during sleep.

Mirror image of dreaming

Whenever we start thinking our eyes are 'parked" and stop taking in information (exactly the same method usee by sleep), to enable Alpha and Beta waves to run your thoughts through to a resolution.
Which leads to the shatteringly simple and obvious conclusion, that during our waking periods, by deliberately recalling memories and running them in a logical sequence, we are mirroring the same function as REM when it re-enacts 'survival' scenarios?
In other words we use our Imagination and although punctuated equilibrium theory may explain Imagination as a sudden and unique mutation. Its process is too similar to REM sleep to be ignored so it is logical to assume that Imagination is simply the result of the mechanical processes used during sleep somehow leaking into our day time activities?

And it happened approximately one hundred thousand years ago, when another 'Big Bang' exploded on the plains of Africa. Suddenly a hominid experienced a new phenomenon; Beta waves started pulling out memories and Alpha waves manipulated them into scenarios during its waking hours. A simply event, which in the beginning may have caused the first Homo sapiens considerable psychological distress, even extreme mental illness. Nevertheless, they not only survived to pass on this new mutation but just as rapidly evolved another feature which is unique to our species, the massive development in our Cerebral Cortex. Purpose built to house and co-ordinate this huge increase in our day-time cognitive activity together they propelled us into a brand new world - the world of Imagination.

Since then Homo imaginus's development has been spectacular, and even though our ability to consciously select and manipulate memories has exploded us like a virulent pathogen onto our moon, we still only stand at the very threshold of our potential. Because Imagination inhabits another dimension, a virtual reality so powerful its limitations are,contradictorily, unimaginable!
It is a universe so vast that it may be infinite and is why it is impossible to predict (Rumsfeld), where we are headed from this,our embryonic, stage. It may be that one day we cross over to exist permanently in its virtual world. As yet nobody knows, but what we do know it that it is indeed possible to look back and trace the unique path, with all its incredible twists and turns, that brought us from the creation of our planet to the very instant we became Homo imaginus and in Part two 'The Journey', we shall attempt to do so.
Sweet Dreams.

The Evolution of Imagination

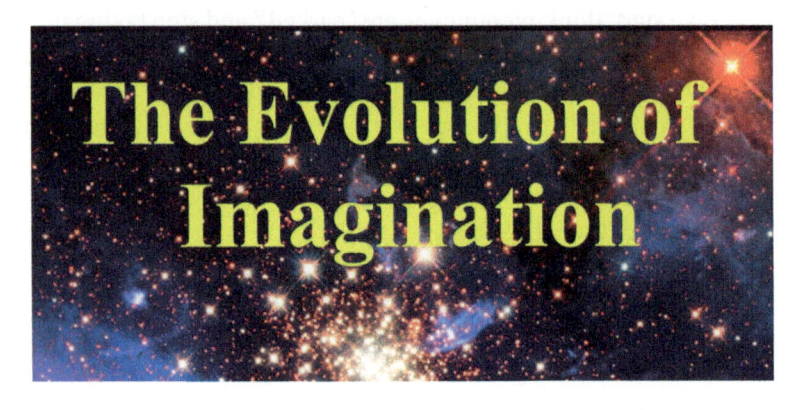

Part 2.

The Journey

The Journey traces the extraordinary steps in the evolution of Imagination – it twists and turns through a series of incredible landscapes that inevitably lead to us, Homo imaginus and in particular, 'The Voice'. The other party in an internal dialogue that constantly articulates our thoughts and ideas which cannot be switched off!

The Journey pinpoints for the first time the very place that complex cells evolved over two billion years ago and documents the incredible series of 'Little Big Bangs' that resulted in the explosion in diversity of life that we know today.

The Journey offers a final proof as to why no other animal on our planet possesses Imagination and comes up with some surprising conclusions about the existence of life, not only in our Solar System and Galaxy, but the Universe.

Further details and pre-order from:

www.evolutionofimagination.com

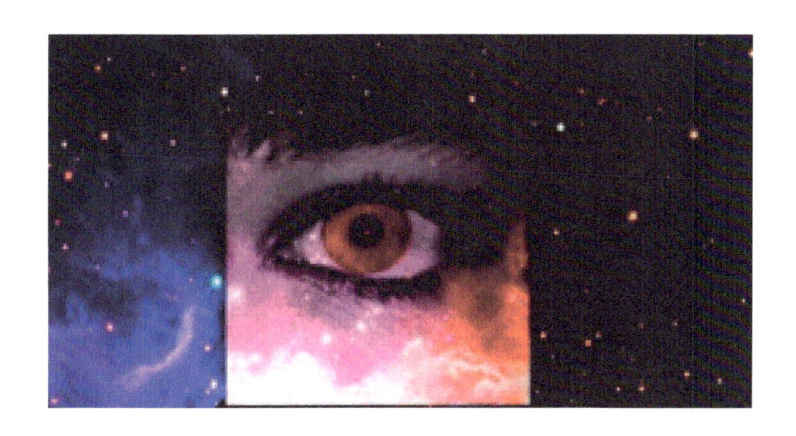

For updates, further information and related links:

www.nightmareofsleep.com

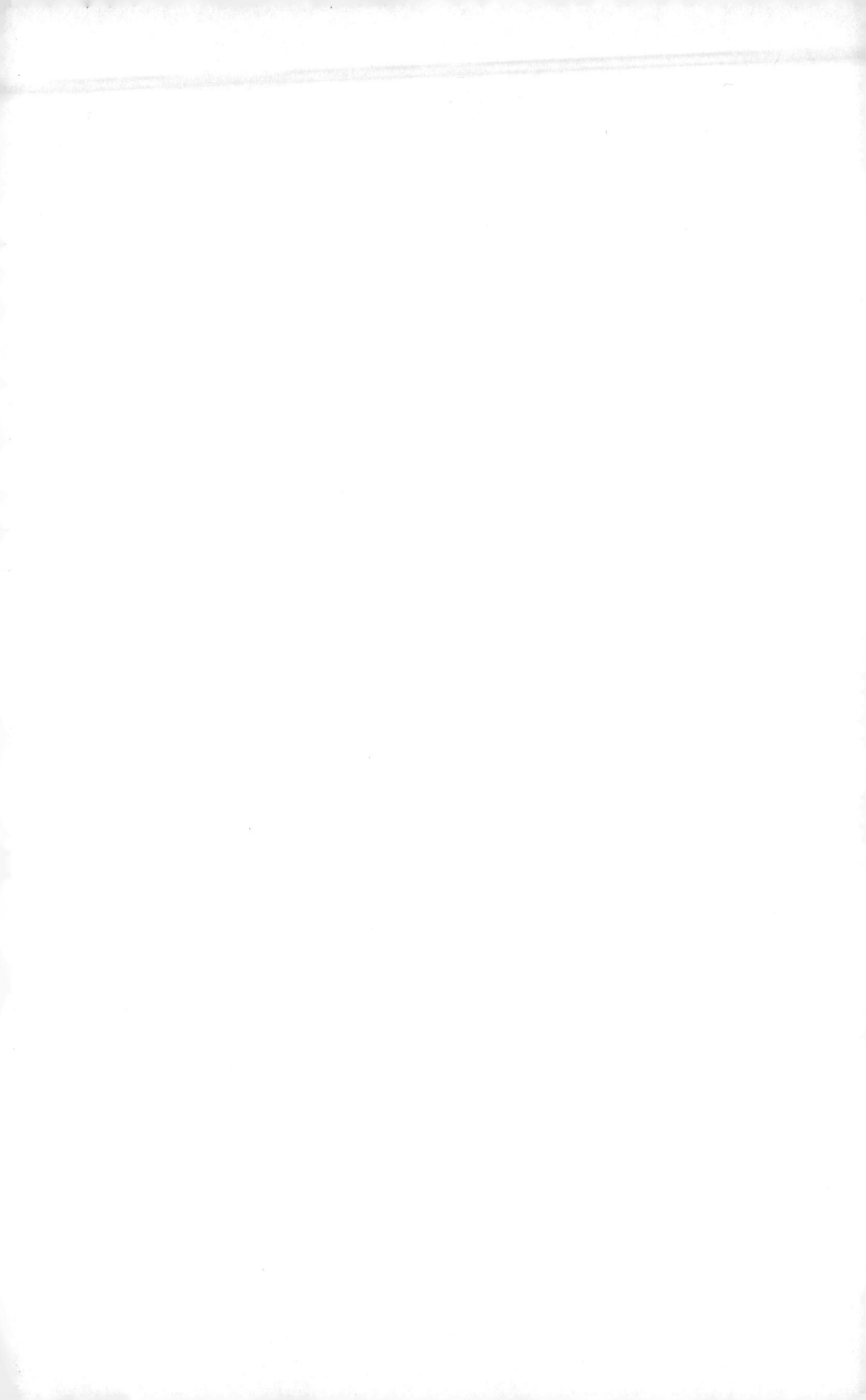

CPSIA information can be obtained at www.ICGtesting.com
Printed in the USA
LVOW011508070313

3411LVUK00013B/28/P

9 781909 465022